Jürgen H.R. THOMAR

RUDOLF BREUSS CANCER CURE
CORRECTLY APPLIED

*This book is dedicated to Rudolf Breuss without **whom I would not have recovered**, and to my dear wife Hertha, without whom I would not have been able to endure the treatment program*

JÜRGEN H.R. Thomar

Correctly applied

RUDOLF BREUSS
CANCER CURE

Original title: Jürgen H.R. Thomar: *Die Krebskur nach Rudolf Breuss richtig gemacht*

GUIDE TO CANCER TREATMENT

I would like to extend my thanks to Mrs. Helene Kleeblatt for her encouraging and dedicated assistance in reshaping this edition into a book which will probably also engage those readers who are critical of empirical therapy.

I would also like to express my gratitude to Professor Dr. Dieter Gebauer who also advocates the Breuss cancer cure and has provided valuable recommendations on the medical aspects of this book.

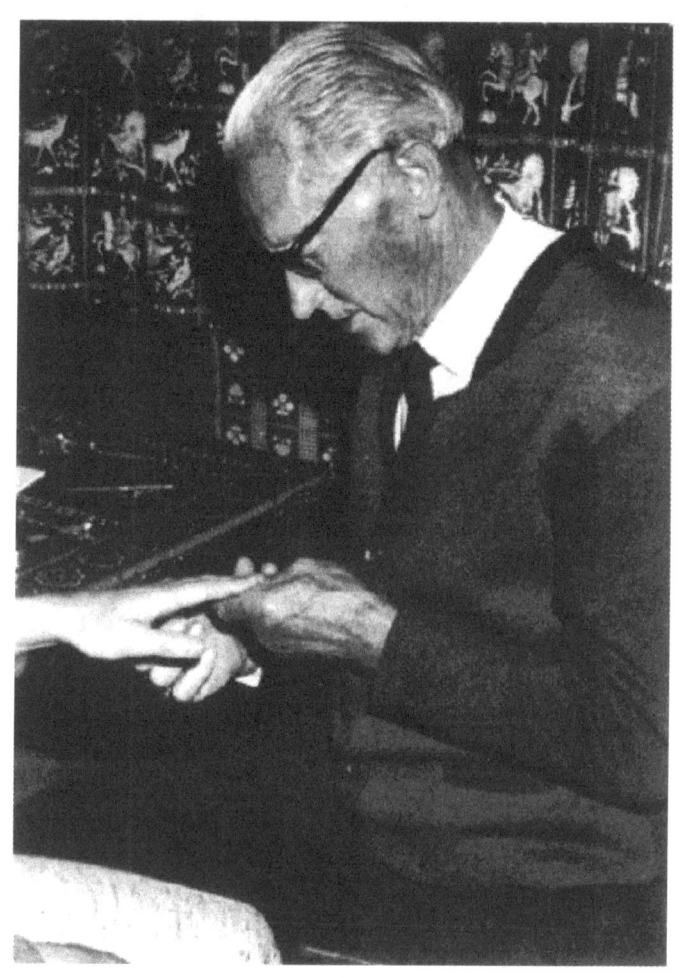

The photograph of Rudolf Breuss diagnosing a patient is courtesy of the Walter Margreiter Publishing House.

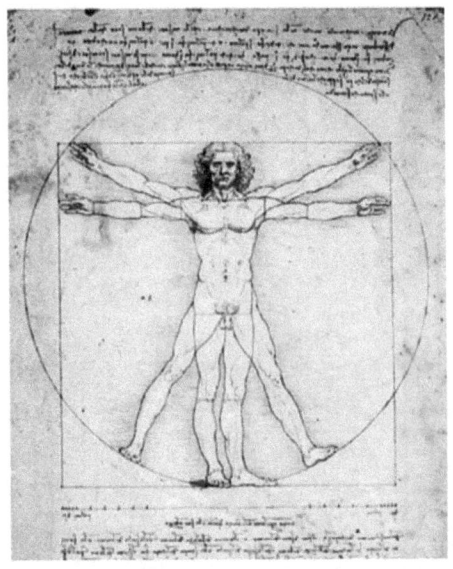

Humans as harmonious beings – human proportions by Leonardo da Vinci – these are the convictions that motivated me to propagate the Breuss Cancer Cure treatment.

Jürgen H.R. Thomar

Important Information for My Readers

What I Am Referring to

The reference document for this guide is Rudolf Breuss' fundamental work "Advice for the Prevention and Natural Treatment of Cancer, Leukemia and Other Seemingly Incurable Diseases", ISBN: 3-00-018407-4, Merk Publishing House, Wangen im Allgäu.

Disclaimer

The author's tips and recommendations offered in this book are intended for informing cancer patients about the proper application of the Breuss Cure treatment. They are not intended to replace the original statements of a naturopath.

In his book, the author does not, either directly or indirectly, offer any medical advice, nor does he prescribe a therapeutic diet without medical consultation.

The author provides no prescriptions in his book; instead, he offers health-related information, which can help you, in cooperation with your doctor, in your quest for health.

By utilizing this information without the consultation with a medical practitioner or your doctor, you engage in self-treatment, which is your human right.

The author assumes no liability for personal injury, property and/or financial loss

© 2015 Thomar

Proofreading: Christina Thomar
Book cover design, interior layout and typesetting:
Jürgen H.R. Thomar

Translation: Task Force Translation Agency, taskforce.com.ua

The author reserves the right to make changes without prior notice and without individual notification of the owners of the previous editions.

All rights reserved. No part of this publication can be distributed, reproduced or transmitted in any form or by any means, electronic or mechanical, including cinema, radio or TV broadcasting, photocopying, recording, or any information storage and retrieval system, without the permission of the author.

First edition – August 2004
Second edition – May 2005
Third edition – January 2008
Fourth edition – January 2011
Fifth edition – April 2014

First edition in English – December 2015

ISBN 978-1511969741

Table of Contents

FOREWORD 19
  PROF. DR. MED., DR.-ING. DIETER GEBAUER

NOTES TO THE 5TH EDITION 21
- GUIDE TO CANCER TREATMENT 21
- AUTHOR PROFILE 21
- PUBLICITY 23
- LITERATURE ON BREUSS 25
- SUMMON THE COURAGE 27

CHAPTER 1
RUDOLF BREUSS –
A PERSON AND NATUROPATHIC PRACTITIONER 28
- HIS PATH IN LIFE 28
- BREUSS JUICE FAST IN THE FIGHT AGAINST CANCER 30
- RUDOLF BREUSS FASTING THERAPY – SIMPLY INGENIOUS 30
- THE TREATMENT IS ALSO HELPFUL IN FIGHTING OTHER ILLNESSES 31
  - □ JOINT INFLAMMATIONS 31
  - □ PULMONARY TUBERCULOSIS 32
  - □ MULTIPLE SCLEROSIS 32
- THE BREUSS MASSAGE 33

CHAPTER 2
HOW I CONQUERED CANCER IN 42 DAYS ... .35
- YOU'VE GOT CANCER 35
- OTHER DIAGNOSTIC PROCEDURES 36
- AGONY OF CHOICE: THE RIGHT THERAPY 37
- REPEAT EXAMINATION: CANCER CAME BACK 38
- THERAPY FAILED. WHAT NEXT? 40
- EXPERTS SUGGEST: TRIPLE THERAPY 40
- A WARNING FROM THE HOSPITAL 42
- MY SALVATION: THE BREUSS CANCER TREATMENT! 42

- How I survived it My Treatment Diary 45
- My Conclusion at the End of the Cancer Treatment. 53
- Cancer Overcome with the Breuss Method 55
- Due to the Breuss Cancer Treatment,
- My Thyroid Has Been Healed! 57
- Weight Loss: Unavoidable Whilst Fasting 58
- How Long Can a Human Fast? 60
- 80 Days without Food Are Probably the Maximum 60
- Science Discovers the Hunger Cure 61

CHAPTER 3
Cancer Treatment 63
- Surgery without a Scalpel 63
- Treatment Directions 64
- Daily Breuss Treatment Plan 65
  - Early morning 65
  - In the morning 66
  - From morning till noon 66
  - At noon 66
  - In the afternoon 66
  - From noon till evening 67
  - In the evening 67
  - Throughout the day 67
  - Additional teas for various types of cancer 68

CHAPTER 4
Differentiated Treatment for
Various Types of Cancer 70
- The scope of cancer treatment:
  from the eyes to the tongue 70
- Treating other types of cancer 79
- Special compresses 80
- Cabbage leaf compress 80
- Hot wraps 82

Table of Contents

CHAPTER 5
SEARCHING FOR THE SOLUTION 85
- FINDING YOUR OWN PATH 85

CHAPTER 6
IMPORTANT TIPS ON THE TREATMENT 93
- BEFORE THE TREATMENT 93
  - ☐ MEDICAL SUPERVISION 93
  - ☐ SPIRITUAL AND MENTAL PREPARATION 95
  - ☐ PHYSICAL PREPARATION 96
    - DRINK A LOT 96
    - EAT EASILY DIGESTIBLE FOODS 97
  - ☐ BOWEL CLEANSING 97
    - GLAUBER'S SALT OR EPSOM SALT 98
    - SAUERKRAUT JUICE 98
    - MUSTARD SEEDS 99
    - ENEMA 99
    - COLON HYDROTHERAPY 99
  - ☐ PREPARATION AT HOME 99
    - SLEEP PLACE INVESTIGATION 99
    - POISON IN YOUR APARTMENT 100
- ORGANIZATIONAL PREPARATION 100
- ARE YOU TOO WEAK FOR THE TREATMENT? 103
- DURING THE TREATMENT 105
  - ☐ BLOOD PRESSURE, SOMETIMES TOO HIGH AND SOMETIMES TOO LOW 105
  - ☐ CONSTIPATION 106
  - ☐ BAD BREATH AND BODY ODOUR 108
    - BAD BREATH 108
    - BODY ODOUR 109
  - ☐ HEADACHE 110
    - INSUFFICIENT BOWEL MOVEMENTS 110
    - NOT DRINKING ENOUGH 110
    - TOO MUCH STRESS 111

Table of Contents

- WITHDRAWAL SYMPTOMS 112
- ☐ OUT IN THE FRESH AIR! 113
- ☐ VEGETABLE JUICE AND ADDITIONAL JUICES 113
- ☐ SMOKING 114
- ☐ EATING AND DRINKING BEYOND MEDICAL
- ☐ DRINKING WATER 114
    - PRESCRIPTIONS 115
- ☐ INJECTIONS, CHEMOTHERAPY, RADIOTHERAPY
    AND DRUGS 115
- ☐ NORMAL WORK DURING CANCER TREATMENT 116
- ☐ CANCER TREATMENT ON THE MOVE 118
- ☐ (SHORT) TRIPS DURING CANCER TREATMENT 119
- ☐ HAPPINESS HORMONES… 120
- AFTER TREATMENT: TAKING CONTROL OF SUCCESS 121
    - ☐ DIAGNOSTIC PROCEDURES 121
    - ☐ DISPUTABLE DIAGNOSTIC PROCEDURES 122
    - ☐ QUESTION AT THE END OF TREATMENT:
        AM I HEALED NOW? 124
    - ☐ TEMPORARY CURE? 125
    - ☐ CONVENTIONAL MEDICINE AVOIDS USING
        THE WORD "CURED" 128
    - ☐ WHAT I DID – AND WHAT I WISH I HAD DONE 128
    - ☐ FAST BREAKING AND READAPTATION 128
        - PRELIMINARY REMARKS 128
        - BREAKING YOUR FAST 130
        - READAPTATION 132
    - ☐ OUR NEW DIET 135
    - ☐ A HEARTH OF YOUR OWN IS WORTH GOLD 137
        DOES THIS PROVERB ALSO APPLY TO MICROWAVE OVENS
        AND INDUCTION COOKERS 137
    - DO INDUCTION STOVES PLACE A PREGNANT WOMAN AND
        FETUS AT RISK? 139
    - ☐ THE TREATMENT IS OVER - KEEP MOVING! 140

Table of Contents

CHAPTER 7
STRENGTHENING YOUR IMMUNE SYSTEM 143
- ☐ FACTORS THAT WEAKEN OUR IMMUNE SYSTEM 143
- ☐ FACTORS THAT STRENGTHEN OUR IMMUNE SYSTEM 145
- ☐ DOES PROTEIN CAUSE HYPERACIDITY? 147
  - ACID-ALKALINE BALANCE 147
  - IS MALNUTRITION TO BLAME? 147
  - TESTING YOUR pH LEVELS 148
  - CONCLUSIONS BASED ON TEST RESULTS 149
  - LESS PROTEIN MEANS MORE HEALTH? 149
  - BEWARE OF A HIGH-PROTEIN
    DIET LEADING TO HYPERACIDITY! 150
- ☐ TIPS FOR HEALTHY EATING 152
  - LESSONS LEARNED FROM FASTING THERAPY 152
  - THE IMPORTANCE OF A FULLY FUNCTIONAL
    METABOLISM 152
  - DON'T EAT IN HASTE! 153
  - STAY HEALTHY AS LONG AS POSSIBLE 153
  - WE ALL HAVE THE POWER TO REDUCE
    THE RISK OF CANCER 154
  - WHAT MUST BE AVOIDED BY ALL MEANS 155
  - REHEATED FOOD 156
  - PROTEIN REVISITED 156
  - HEALTHY FOOD 158
- ☐ TIPS ON DRINKING "GOOD WATER" 159
  - TAP WATER
    THE MOST REGULATED FOODSTUFF (?) 159
  - WORLD WATER QUALITY ASSESSMENT 162
  - IS MINERAL WATER THE BEST QUALITY WATER? 164
  - DISTILLED WATER 166
  - WHAT WATER DO THE THOMARS DRINK? 167
  - WATER PURIFICATION FILTERS 168
  - PURPOSE AND MECHANISM OF REVERSE OSMOSIS 169
  - CLEANING WATER

Table of Contents

- with Advanced Filtration Technology 170
  - Advantages of Such Equipment 170
  - What's in Our Drinking Water? 171
  - So, What Is "Good Water"? 173
- Mothballs, Water Veins and Earth Radiation 173
  - Mothballs 173
  - Water Veins and Earth Radiation 174
  - Do We Need Dietary Supplements Nowadays? ...176
  - And What Do We Need
    to Know about Dietary Supplements? 176
  - Isn't Regular Food Good Enough Anymore? 176
  - Why Doesn't Our Body Get All the Necessary
    Nutrients, Though We Are Made
    to Believe Otherwise? 177
  - The main reason is mineral depletion of soil 177
  - Other Reasons for Lack of Vital Nutrients 181
  - In Common Foods 181
  - Eating Less Does Not Mean
    Requiring Fewer Nutrients 181
  - Ready-Made Food 181
  - Microwave Oven 182
  - Stress Factors 182
  - Today We Are Hungry Despite Being
    "Chock-Full" 182
  - Conclusions to Be Drawn Personally 182

CHAPTER 8
The Special Juice 185
- Treatment Cornerstones 185
- Shall I Press Juice Myself or Buy Ready-made Juice? 185
  - What Are the Benefits of Juice Pressed at Home? .185
  - What Are the Benefits of Ready-made Juice? 186
- How You Should Drink the Juice 187
- Making Your Own Vegetable Juice 188

Table of Contents

- On the Subject of Potato 190
- If You Don't Like Vegetable Juice (Anymore) 190
  - Vegetable Juice with Orange 191
  - Vegetable Juice with Sauerkraut 191
  - Vegetable Juice with Lemon 192

CHAPTER 9
Special Broths and Tinctures 194
- Important Components of Effective Treatment 194
  - Onion Broth 194
  - Broth of Bean Pods 195
  - Hawthorn Tincture 196

CHAPTER 10
Special Teas 197
- Another Treatment Cornerston 197
- Infusions (Brews, Teas) to Be Taken
  for <u>All</u> Cancer Types 199
  - Kidney Tea 199
  - Marigold Te 200
  - Sage Tea 200
  - Cranesbill (Herb Robert) Tea 202
  - Special Tea Mix 203
- Additional Teas for <u>Specific</u> Cancer Types 205
  - Eyebright Tea 205
  - Valerian Tea 205
  - Pimpernel Tea 206
  - Potatoes' Skin Tea 206
  - Lemon Balm Tea 206
  - Celandine Tea 207
  - Silver Lady's Mantle and Lady's Mantle Tea 207
  - Willow Herb Tea 208
  - Wormwood or Centaury Tea 208
  - Wormwood Tea 208

Table of Contents

- ☐ Tea Preparation is a Matter of Organization 209
- ☐ If the Teas No Longer Taste Good 212
  - ☐ Tea with Lemon 212
  - ☐ Teas with Various Strength....................................212

CHAPTER 11
Cancer Treatment Shopping List....................213
- Arrangements First! 213
  - ☐ How Much Juice Vegetables Provide....................213
  - ☐ Posttreatment Use of Leftover Herbal Tea Leaves...213
- Treatment Shopping List 214
  - ☐ Problems with buying herbal medicines?...................219
  - ☐ Can't find Ligusticum mutellina? 219
  - ☐ Can't find Bio-Strath (Strath) / PK-Strath?..........221
  - ☐ Can't find a herbal tea or vegetable juice? 221

CHAPTER 12
The Breuss Total Cancer Treatment Undergoes Clinical Trial 222
- What I wish for at the time of writing........................222
- The oncology report by Professor Douwes, MD: «*How reasonable is fasting therapy for treating cancer patients?*» 223
  - ☐ Procedure..225
  - ☐ Medical supervision 226
  - ☐ Results 226
  - ☐ Conclusions 229
  - ☐ Discussion...230
- Feedback from conventional medical community 231
  - ☐ There is some progress in the case! 233
  - ☐There is some progress in the case! 233

Table of Contents

CHAPTER 13
CURRENT CANCER STATISTICS **235**
- NEW CANCER CASES 235
- NEW CANCER CASES WORLDWIDE 235
- NEW CANCER CASES IN GERMANY 236
  - MOST COMMON CANCERS IN MALES 237
  - MOST COMMON CANCERS IN FEMALES 237
  - CHILDHOOD CANCERS 237
  - CANCER DIAGNOSIS 238
- PROSTATE CANCER, SCOURGE AMONG MEN 241
  - PREVENTIVE CANCER SCREENING 241
- BREAST CANCER, SCOURGE AMONG WOMEN 242
  - EARLY CANCER SCREENING 243
- COLORECTAL CANCER, SCOURGE AMONG MEN
  AND WOMEN 245
  - EARLY CANCER SCREENING 245

CHAPTER 14
FOR THE BENEFIT OF THE PEOPLE? **248**
- QUO VADIS, CANCER TREATMENT 248
- FASTING CANCER TREATMENT STARTS THE THERAPY! 249
- 40% OF ALL CANCER CASES CAN BE PREVENTED! 249
- THE ROLE OF THE PATIENT 250

CHAPTER 15
I HAVE A VISION **252**
- MAY WISHES COME TRUE 252
- MY PERSONAL WISH AT
  THE END OF THE BOOK 254

Table of Contents

APPENDIX 1 DAILY SCHEDULE 256
APPENDIX 2 DAY 35 259
APPENDIX 3 I DID IT!!! A MODEL FORM 261
APPENDIX 4 QUESTIONNAIRE FOR COLLECTING THE BREUSS THERAPY-BASED CANCER HEALING TESTIMONIALS 263
   DATA SHEET FOR COLLECTING THE BREUSS THERAPY-BASED CANCER HEALING TESTIMONIALS 265
APPENDIX 5 TEA LABELS 266
APPENDIX 6 BIBLIOGRAPHY 267
APPENDIX 7 ADDRESS DIRECTORY 273
APPENDIX 8 SUBJECT INDEX..278

Foreword by
Dr. Dieter Gebauer, Professor, Doctor of Medicine, Doctor of Engineering

Rudolf Breuss, with his juice fasting program of cancer treatment, has developed a surprisingly effective form of therapy, which for decades has proved to be helpful for many people suffering from cancer.

The Rudolf Breuss juice fasting treatment requires determination and self-discipline on the part of the patient. This treatment cannot give a promise of healing; however, in my view it represents a promising supportive therapy used to treat various types of cancer.

My previous research has demonstrated that every single patient I know of, everyone who underwent the 42-day Breuss cure treatment, has at least markedly improved his health. Most cases go so far as to cure a tumor or cancer.

So far there has hardly been any data on how the Breuss cure treatment works. This fact prevents many physicians and naturopaths from recommending it to their patients. At the same time, during the Breuss cure treatment, sound medical care, including necessary examinations, is as **important** as during other therapeutic measures. Furthermore, holistic therapy based on cooperation between all medical fields, including those related to adjunctive care, is of utmost significance in healing cancer patients.

Mr. Thomar, with his book "Rudolf Breuss Cancer Cure Correctly Applied", deserves credit for providing systemic description of the treatment, thus developing a guide to the Breuss Cancer Cure.

Foreword of Dr. Dieter Gebauer, Professor, Doctor of Medicine, Doctor of Engineering

This book is a major contribution to understanding the Breuss Cancer Cure that provides recommendations on its successful implementation – I wish it great success!

Gmund / Ostin am Tegernsee, December 2007

Dr. Dieter Gebauer, Professor, Doctor of Medicine, Doctor of Engineering

ACKNOWLEDGEMENT AND GRATITUDE TO RUDOLF BREUSS

⌘

GUIDE TO CANCER TREATMENT

This book represents my gratitude to Rudolf Breuss who died in 1990 at the age of 91, and who helped me with his extensive knowledge and experience to defeat cancer. With this book I would also like to make my contribution to promoting the Breuss cancer cure so that one day this treatment – as has long been recommended by experts like Prof. Dr. med. Friedrich Douwes and Dr. Veronica Carstens - would be implemented <u>before</u> each use of scalpel and radiation therapy, and not <u>after</u> it, when it is too late. Unfortunately, today the Breuss cancer cure is often used as a last-ditch effort when the patient is "untreatable" (the verdict which is too often and prematurely made by oncologists, instead of offering patients hope and helping them), abandoned by conventional medicine and sent home to die. But even then it can be not too late to turn to the Breuss cancer cure, as is shown in the Oncology Report in Chapter 12.

Author Profile

I, Jürgen H.R. Thomar, was born 1938 in Magdeburg; in 2001 I was diagnosed with prostate cancer. A year after undergoing conventional medical treatment at a university hospital, that is in 2002, I was diagnosed with recurrent cancer, or remained uncured of my first cancer

Since the triple therapy which was designed for me after numerous examinations that followed, was not been scientifically

Acknowledgement And Gratitude To Rudolf Breuss

documented, and I was to become a guinea pig, I turned away from conventional oncology and resorted to naturopathy.

Given that I was a lay person in terms of medical knowledge – I was a retired staff officer and later a managing director of an IT-company – I found a book to help me, "Natural Treatment of Cancer, Leukemia and Other Seemingly Incurable Diseases" by Rudolf Breuss, a well-known healer, naturopath and folk medicine expert from Bludenz in Austria.

Spring 2004, I applied and followed the Breuss Cancer Cure treatment and was completely cured of cancer. As proven by all subsequent examinations, the treatment was a complete success. I am healthy again.

After that, as a mark of gratitude to Rudolf Breuss, I created the website www.breuss-kur.de which has generated immense interest worldwide: so far, it has received over 200, 000 visitors. And their number is growing by the day…

I handed over my company to younger hands and devoted myself fully to fighting cancer and advocating Breuss and the Breuss cancer cure.

My contribution as the author of "Rudolf Breuss Cancer Cure Correctly Applied", as experts say, is to add a practical dimension to the Breuss cure treatment and in so doing to create an easily comprehensible and well-defined guide to implementing the treatment. My books are considered as basic manuals to successful application of the Breuss cancer cure. It is noteworthy that both the original edition of Breuss' book "Natural Treatment of Cancer, Leukemia and Other Seemingly Incurable Diseases" (page 162) and its newly revised edition "The Breuss Cancer Cure" (p. 6), explicitly recommend my book as a manual.

Acknowledgement And Gratitude To Rudolf Breuss

By the way, I live in a place where others come for a vacation, in the Bodensee region, and I have also written the books "Rudolf Breuss Fasting Therapy – Simply Ingenious" and "Practical Guide to Breuss Treatment: Experience, Tips and Recommendations" that have been translated into French. My work "Rudolf Breuss Cancer Cure Correctly Applied" has also been translated into Albanian and Slovenian.

Publicity

If you wish to advocate this therapy, you can't keep it to yourself. There is a need to make it public. On the one hand, I perform this task through my books and the website. On the other hand, it is necessary to engage the media. This objective, given its massive global reach, should be pursued on a continuing basis.

Following my presentation on October 29, 2010 on the German TV channel SWR Fernsehen in a panel discussion with the presenter Mr. Wieland Backes under the topic "Food – an Enemy or Elixir of Life?" dealing with the Breuss cancer cure and its successful application, Radio ENERGY, BERLIN 103,4 held an interview with me that was broadcast nation-wide, also on the subject of cancer and naturopathy.

And finally in summer 2012, KRfilm Berlin made a documentary about a patient who was healed of breast cancer, under the title "Dying is Cancelled – Life with Cancer".

The film was broadcast nation-wide on September 4, 2012 on the SAT.1 channel. It was a significant contribution to the promotion of the Breuss treatment. The editorial staff of the KRfilm studio describes their documentary as follows:
"The diagnosis of 'cancer' is always a shock. In a single second, it completely changes the life of the patient and his or her family members.

Acknowledgement And Gratitude
To Rudolf Breuss

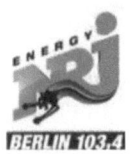

This film describes the fate of three women and their families who had to learn to live with this horrible diagnosis. The authors show the life of three mothers in their families. It deals with hope, fear, love, death and trust. 'Dying is Cancelled – Life with Cancer' is also the film about three strong women. In their struggle against cancer they were forced to concentrate on the essentials".

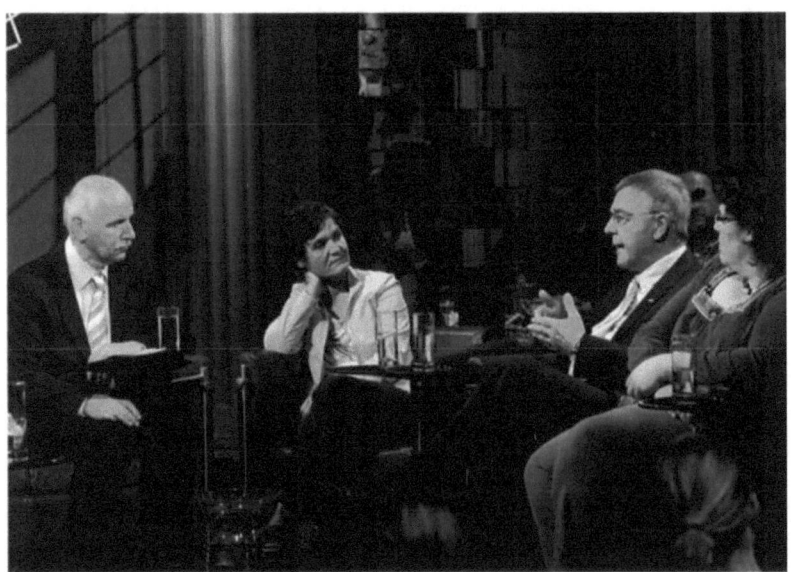

Photo: The author with the presenter Wieland Backes in the NACHTCAFE studio of the SWR studio, discussing the topic "Food – an Enemy or Elixir of Life?"

My remark: here we are focusing on the fate of Silke Seifert who has overcome cancer through Breuss treatment. The two other women tried to beat cancer with conventional medicine.

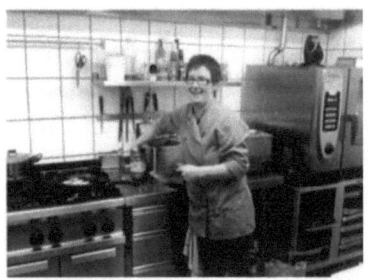

Silke Seifert in her kitchen

Acknowledgement And Gratitude To Rudolf Breuss

The film editors continue: «*3 years ago Silke Seifert (47) was diagnosed with breast cancer. Initially she was treated by the application of drugs. When she is informed of the date of mastectomy, she refuses any further treatment. She undergoes a 6-week fasting program that restricts her to exclusively juices and teas and removes toxins from her body; this is designed to deprive cancer of its nourishment. And in six weeks her cancer is indeed gone. Today Silke Seifert has regular blood tests, to control her values. She has completely changed her diet – no sugar, pork, no cigarettes. She says: "Never before have I felt as healthy as now!"*

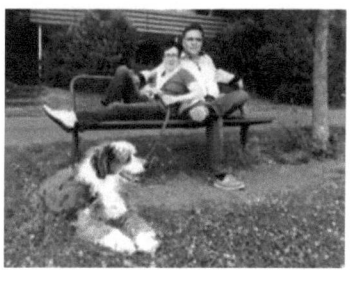

We finally got over the hump. Now it is time to relax. Silke and Uwe Seifert.

This film undoubtedly deserves attention

Literature on Breuss

During my lectures, seminars and also in discussions I often discovered that many families have the little yellow book "Natural Treatment of Cancer, Leukemia and Other Seemingly Incurable Diseases" by Rudolf Breuss. It is no wonder since this book has sold more than one million copies worldwide.

When I start asking questions, it turns out that almost nobody has read this book to the end. Seldom have I met people who went through the Breuss treatment, or their family members who did read the book. Why is that?

The reason is that Breuss – when asked to write down the most important features of his cancer treatment to save them from

Acknowledgement And Gratitude To Rudolf Breuss

oblivion – was of quite an advanced age. Following that, his records were published; however, they have never been edited, externally compiled or adapted.

The same happened to me: I raced through the book and concluded that it would be difficult to undergo a course of cancer treatment in a way described by the author in the Chapter "Directions for the Treatment" and specified in the Chapter "How the Total Cancer Treatment Works". The author gave numerous tips, recommendations and also prohibitions throughout the book, instead of summarizing them in the chapters above.

In order to carry out my own treatment in the proper manner, I have thoroughly studied Breuss' book and highlighted, summarized and structured the most crucial information, as Rudolf Breuss writes, "The treatment can only fail in case when my instructions are not strictly adhered to in all aspects". For me this was a decisive impulse to bring my elaborations on the treatment into a systematized and structured form – as a step-by-step guide - because I was not going to fast for nothing!

In the spring of 2005, the first edition of my book came out, still under the title "Rudolf Breuss Total Cancer Treatment Correctly Applied". The book was based on the original work of Breuss' "Natural Treatment of Cancer, Leukemia and Other Seemingly Incurable Diseases" published by the Merk Publishing House. Today, I know that there are three books on the market written by the author:

1. The publication above in its original edition.
2. The book "The Breuss Cancer Cure" published by the Walter Margreiter Mail-Order Bookshop and Publishing House specializing in Breuss' works.
3. The book "Natural Treatment of Cancer, Leukemia and

Acknowledgement And Gratitude To Rudolf Breuss

Other Seemingly Incurable Diseases" – co-authored by R. Breuss and Dr. C. Moermann, AURUM/Kamphausen Publishing House.

Summon the Courage

In conclusion, I would like to urge all cancer patients to gather their courage and help themselves. I am convinced that each of us has only one life.

To take responsibility for it, incorporate the experience of others and then make the right decisions for yourself, is certainly a good route!

Isn't it worth trying to beat cancer with 42 days of self-discipline?

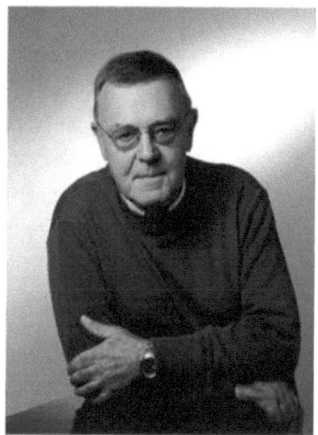

May my progress report help you to be strong!

Jürgen H.R. Thomar

Chapter 1

Rudolf Breuss – a Person and Naturopathic Practitioner

✤

His Path in Life

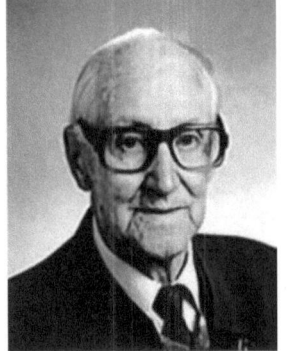

Rudolf Breuss (1899 – 1990) was born on June 24, 1899 in the Austrian town of Feldkirch (federal state Vorarlberg) and attended school there. He grew up together with three siblings. At the age of 14, after leaving school, he began working in a bakery. Two years later the young Breuss moved to work in the telegraph office of Feldkirch.

During World War I, he was inducted into the army and sent to the front in South Tyrol as an artilleryman. But there he fell seriously ill, and after treatment in a military hospital in Innsbruck was discharged from military service. After his return to civilian life, Breuss found employment as a lineman at the telegraph office in Bludenz. In 1920, he married Maria Neyer. They had three daughters and a son.

In 1924, his poor health caused by the war prevented Breuss from carrying out his plan of emigrating overseas.

His health situation, however, awoke his interest in naturopathy. The starting point for this was pastor Kneipp's preaching which

Chapter 1 - Rudolf Breuss – a Person and Naturopathic Practitioner

Breuss continuously tested on himself. Over time, he became familiar with other naturopathic practices and established himself as an iridologist and natural medicine practitioner.

Breuss was also an outstanding inventor: during his time as an industrial electrician at the Innerebner & Meyer construction company in Bludenz, he obtained 6 patents on inventions.

On June 20, 1949, Breuss started working at Vorarlberger power plant as an electrician and worked there until his retirement at the end of 1962. From this time on, he devoted his life to treating the sick and advocating naturopathy.

He tirelessly developed and tested his fasting cure, which consisted of freshly pressed juices and various herbal teas. Using this methodology, Rudolf Breuss cured, by his own estimate, several thousand people suffering from cancer and leukemia, many of whom had been given up by conventional physicians as having no hope. Numerous medical certificates and letters of gratitude confirm this fact.

This fact brought him not only recognition – many of his former patients became his friends. The managing director of a print shop in the town of Wangen im Allgäu whose wife was cured of cancer by Breuss, offered the aged Breuss to write down and publish his method of treatment. Thus, in 1978, they published the booklet "Natural Treatment of Cancer, Leukemia and Other Seemingly Incurable Diseases", millions of copies of which have now been sold worldwide. Up till now, this book has been printed in the Walchner print shop (now "Süd" print shop) in Wangen im Allgäu.

In 1982, Rudolf Breuss managed to apply his juice fasting cure in a hospital of conventional medicine – read more in Chapter 12.
In May 1990 Rudolf Breuss fell ill and died two weeks later at the age of 91.

The handing down of his knowledge through distribution of his book all over the world keeps his legacy alive.

Breuss Juice Fast in the Fight Against Cancer

Breuss explains his success by the fact that the cancer cells are "starved to death" through the juice fast. In fact, this method supports the patients with raw vegetable juices without stressing the body, using the indisputable healing effect of fasting therapy. Extending the fasting period to 42 days can consolidate the successful results.

In 2007, I had the opportunity to experience how effective a determined and consistent fasting can be: while visiting an acquaintance of mine, a reputable doctor from Bavaria, I heard her incredible life story: Mrs. P., Dr. med., was diagnosed with cancer 25 years ago. She had never heard of Breuss, however, she knew about the remedial powers of fasting. So, for 48 (!) days she went without eating and drank <u>nothing</u> but pure water.

The lady lost a lot of weight, reaching an incredible 25 kg. At that time she was pregnant and during the fasting period gave birth to a baby. The baby-girl was born healthy and developed quite adequately; today, she is 25 years old. Mrs. P., upon completion of her fast, was healed of cancer, and so far the disease has never relapsed.

Rudolf Breuss Fasting Therapy – Simply Ingenious

Thus, long-term fasting can be very effective. However, the Breuss cancer cure fast is not so strict, and not so difficult to get through, since the Breuss fasting includes a good deal of supporting foods and drinks.

Chapter 1 - Rudolf Breuss – a Person and Naturopathic Practitioner

The meeting with Mrs. P. was a decisive reason for me for taking up fasting therapy as an effective treatment, collecting all available knowledge about this therapy, comparing my experience with that of others and, ultimately, for writing a book about it (see p. 85). In the meantime, I had personally been exposed to the Breuss strict fasting for 103 days (distributed over several treatments in the last years).

By the way, I think it would be unjust to limit the Breuss treatment "only" to fighting cancer. This method is able to accomplish much more than "only" to fight cancer. In my book about the fasting therapy I come to that in greater detail.

The Treatment Is Also Helpful in Fighting Other Illnesses

"My juice therapy", writes Rudolf Breuss ,*"fights not only cancer, but also the following illnesses:*

Joint Inflammation

Joint inflammations as arthritis (inflammatory joint disease), arthrosis (degenerative joint inflammation), coxarthrosis (disease of the hip joint), osteoporosis (bone decalcification) and spondylarthrosis (arthrosis of the dorsal and lumbar vertebrae): all these conditions require no more than a three-week juice therapy, but it has to be undergone with strict adherence to the instructions, no less strict than those for treating cancer, including taking kidney and sage tea". Should you want to undergo the treatment for the full 42 days, continues Breuss, it certainly will not hurt you; on the contrary, it will rid your body of any possible cancer cells.

The proper way to carry out the treatment in case of joint inflammations is described in my book "Rudolf Breuss Fasting

Therapy – Simply Ingenious" (see Bibliography). The "prescribed" baths turned out truly beneficial for my joints and me

Pulmonary Tuberculosis

The cancer cure described is effective not only for joint inflammations, but also for pulmonary tuberculosis. This disease requires a regular cancer cure. Additionally, you should daily take one teaspoonful of broadleaf plantain seeds with some tea. Broadleaf plantain seeds are sold in pharmacies as Indian plantago seeds.

Multiple Sclerosis

Here is what Breuss' original book says about multiple sclerosis:
"Breathing exercises as prescribed for high blood pressure, but in this case they should be done 20-30 times a day, each time lasting 5-10 minutes. In addition, it would be useful to carry out my 42-day fast with vegetable juices and herbal teas as in the case of cancer. In this way I have so far successfully cured around 30 patients who consulted me, some of them were from so far away as Australia. These 30 people had the same symptoms as in a case of real multiple sclerosis. In the case of real multiple sclerosis, one or several nerve fibers become cut, thus making the disease incurable".

Below, with the author's permission, I quote a personal letter which Breuss wrote on September 28, 1985, at the age of 86, to a lady I knew:
«...*You should drink kidney tea for three weeks. Whenever possible, drink sage tea. Then carry out my juice treatment program as in the case with cancer. For a week, in addition to food, take about half a bottle (or up to a bottle) of my vegetable juice a day. Drink it slowly, about 10 minutes before each meal, some 1/16 litre. And only after this week when the body is accustomed to the juice, start the total treatment. However,* **the most important thing** *is to do breathing exercises exactly as they*

Chapter 1 - Rudolf Breuss – a Person and Naturopathic Practitioner

are prescribed for high blood pressure (my remark: this is described in detail in Breuss' original book).

In multiple sclerosis, only the motor nerve of legs or hands is blocked. This causes paralysis. If patients adhere strictly to all these prescriptions, they can recover in 7 weeks, which I wish them with all my heart. All the 30 persons whom this method of mine has cured so far, in reality had only pseudosclerosis.

If a nerve is torn and the patient is paralyzed, the condition cannot be cured since it really is multiple sclerosis. When there is a block in the brain, the symptoms are the same as those of real multiple sclerosis".

The Breuss Massage

Breuss became renowned not only for his juice and tea therapy, but also for his methods of treating intervertebral disk disorders. His technique of "painless spinal alignment therapy" is used today by many therapists and gains more and more circulation, publicity and popularity.

In conjunction with the Dorn-therapy, the Breuss massage – also known as gentle massage – is literally designed to be made prior to the rather painful Dorn-therapy. Given the fact that I have studied both methods, I would take the liberty to pass judgment in this way.

Rudolf Breuss said that with his spinal therapy, he helped than 7,200 patients to rid of their back ailments.

In Salem, close to my hometown where I got into the subject of Breuss (you'll learn about that later), I got to know the healer Gerhard Kerber in 2005. He was not only a profound expert on Breuss treatment. He showed my wife and I an authentic video

Chapter 1 - Rudolf Breuss -
a Person and Naturopathic Practitioner

film on the techniques of the Breuss massage* produced by the naturopath himself. Mr. Kerber also practices this massage entirely in the spirit of Rudolf Breuss.

You will find Mr. Kerber's address in the address directory (Appendix). You can also learn the Breuss massage in the training center of the Breuss-Dorn-Fleig spine therapy in Wehr (also in the address directory).

≈

---

*) The merit of professional production of this historic film goes to Mr. Michael Rau, from the training center for Breuss and Dorn (address in the Appendix). Interested parties can purchase the film.

Chapter 2
How I Conquered Cancer in 42 Days ...
You've Got Cancer

⌘

As a follow-up to the routine examination I underwent in autumn 2001, at the beginning of 2002, apart from rectal palpation in the urology department, I had a blood test taken – a PSA[1]-test. Outcome: the PSA level was 11.0 ng/ml, diagnosis: prostate cancer!

0-4 ng/ml **PSA** Normal value	>4-10 ng/ml **PSA** Grey area	>10 ng/ml **PSA** Possible carcinoma	11,0 ng/ml **PSA** My PSA value

*) Depending on the patient's age, possible carcinoma can be suspected even at 2 ng/ml.

1)   Determination of the PSA level
Here is what urologists say about the PSA:
PSA = Prostate-specific antigen, protein produced by the male prostate gland (the prostate). The disputed PSA value (see p. 122, section "Taking Control of Success: Diagnostic Procedures") is measured in cases of suspected and existing prostate cancer.
It can also be checked regularly in the framework of annual prostate cancer screening. In case of existing prostate cancer, the PSA value is regularly controlled in order to monitor cancer growth and to measure the success of the therapy.
(Source: the European Association of Urology guidelines, the German Association of Urology guidelines).
You should also know what experts think of the PSA value:
The scientific ournalist Dr. Klaus Koch dwells on the PSA problem:
"The test is not fully adequate because of its high false positive rate". (Ed.: it means the patient is healthy but was falsely identifi d as sick). According to the "Deutsches Ärzteblatt" (German Medical Journal) of 2006 this rate is 75% (Ed.: it means that 75% of patients despite the negative test result are healthy!). It makes the test not only pointless but also dangerous: the psychological impact on misdiagnosed men is enormous".
In my opinion, the PSA test is not advisable. I trust other diagnostic methods (see p. 121)

The "prostate cancer" diagnosis hit me like a bolt of lightning – I never expected that!

My brain reeled at the news, wondering:
- Why me?
- Didn't I quit smoking 11 years ago?
- Didn't I try to avoid stress?
- What do I have to do to cope with this message?
- Can I live with this diagnosis?
- If I can, then for how long?
- What am I to do?
- How much time do I have for this?
- What are my chances of recovery?
- Do I have any chances at all?

Other Diagnostic Procedures

The biopsy and ultrasound examination I underwent revealed adenocarcinoma (a malignant tumor that germinates in the glandular parts of the mucous membrane of an organ), grades G1 to G2.

By the way, more than 95% of all prostate cancers are adenocarcinomas (so-called malignant tumors).

My Gleason score[2] (a unit of measuring the malignancy of cancer and its aggressiveness) was 2+2=4. Since there are 5 Gleason grades, the Gleason score can vary between 2 (1+1) and 10 (5+5).

---

2)   *The American pathologist Donald F. Gleason in 1966 devised the scale of 1 through 5 to grade the degree of malignancy of prostatic carcinoma. The grading is made on the basis of the findings of the microscopic examination.*
To obtain a Gleason score, the dominant (prevalent) pattern is added to the second most prevalent pattern of tumor tissue samples. The score is always determined in conformity with the model: Gleason score 1 + score 2 = sum of both scores (Source: Wikipedia)

Chapter 2 - How I Conquered Cancer in 42 Days …

Prostate carcinomas with Gleason grades of 1 to 3 (that is, score 2 to 6) are usually slow-growing tumors not aggressive in nature. With Gleason grade 4, as in my case, there is a considerably higher probability that the tumor will display more aggressive behaviour. For details, see the graph below.

The results of the examination of tissue samples (biopsies) not only confirmed prostate cancer, but also showed that the cancer was becoming too aggressive.

To specify the diagnosis and control the PSA level, a CT was performed 14 days later. The result: 9.16 ng/ml, that is, somewhat lower than two weeks ago, but still too high.

4 days later, the radiotherapy performed at the university hospital diagnosed a PSA level of 9.2 ng/ml and the Gleason score at the same level of 2+2=4.

Thus, the CT and a repeat blood test confirmed the dreadful diagnosis: prostate cancer.

So, the question arose of how to choose the mode of treatment that would best suit me.

Agony of Choice: the Right Therapy

As a private patient, I was offered the following options:

- radical surgery (removing the entire organ – prostate),
- external radiotherapy, or
- internal radiotherapy (brachytherapy).

I opted for the relatively new and promising (according to physicians, its success rate is about 95%) brachytherapy (from the Greek word brachys, meaning "short-distance"). It is one of the forms of radiotherapy where a radiation source is placed in the patient's body inside the cancer affected area or next to it. Radioactive seeds are implanted directly into the prostate.

The operation was conducted in spring 2002 in the radiotherapy and urology department of a university hospital. The findings of the repeat examination evidenced the success of the therapy: the PSA level of 1.1 ng/ml was exceptionally low.

It was a cause for celebration!

Repeat Examination: Cancer Came Back

One repeat examination conducted in spring 2003 brought sobering news: the cancer came back again (or was still there).

The PSA level rose again to 1.5 ng/ml.

In autumn 2003, the examination performed by the pathology department revealed a higher Gleason score: from the original 2+2=4 it rose to **4+4=8**, that is, it reached the second highest level.

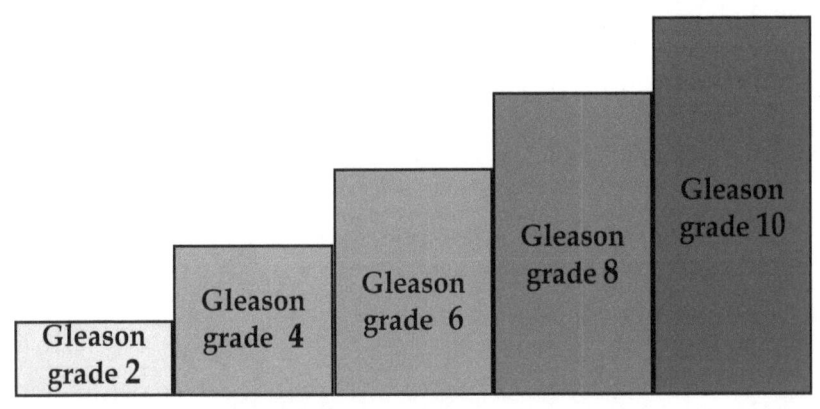

The Gleason score from 2 to 10

Thus, the cancer was indeed back again, and it became more aggressive!

Brachytherapy did not help me!

Therapy Failed. What Next?

After further examinations and intensive discussions with physicians, I was offered the following treatment options developed by conventional medicine:

- **Radical surgery (removing the entire organ – prostate)**
  A detailed analysis of this therapy outlined the following picture (at that time): there is a 50% risk that the cancer will not be totally removed (consequently, the cancer will grow and the operation will be useless). Moreover, radical surgery bears a 50% risk of such a miserable condition as incontinence, so that I would have to wear diapers. In the worst case, as a result of this therapy I would have been a diaper wearer for no longer than some 3 years, which was how long I had to live.

- **External radiotherapy**
  Here, the radiation I had already received through brachytherapy, had to be taken into consideration

- **Repeat brachytherapy**
  In this case, just as well, it would be necessary to take into consideration the radiation I had already received through my first brachytherap

- **Hormone therapy**
  Not very desirable therapy since it can damage masculinity and male hormonal health.

Experts Suggest: Triple Therapy

The experts of the university hospital recommended to me the following therapy as the one offering best chances of success – as viewed by conventional medicine:

Chapter 2 - How I Conquered Cancer in 42 Days ...

1. First, **hormone therapy** over the next two years (with far-reaching consequences for sexual life)

2. Subsequently, 6 weeks after the start of the hormone therapy - **external radiotherapy** for about 6 weeks.

3. Finally - repeat **brachytherapy**, very precisely targeted at the two remaining "hotspots" (cancerous tumors) in the right and left sides of the prostate.

Given the fact that almost half a year had passed after the last examination, this surgery had to be preceded by yet another examination using advanced medical diagnostic equipment (choline-PET-CT) / choline positron emission tomography, in order to shed more light on the situation.

The result of the examination performed on February 23, 2004, said: my PSA level was 1.7 ng/ml. It was in fact not yet a cause for concern, although the actual increase compared with its original value amounted to 70%. But the Gleason score remained at the said 4+4=8.

The cancer (I never wanted either to think or say "my cancer" as the cancerous tumor was not mine, it did not belong to me, it was an extraneous body inside me!) reached the second most aggressive level, turning, so to speak, from a "peaceful pet" into a "ferocious tiger", as it is sometimes said - a little bit offhand - among oncologists.

Thus, a lot of time had been wasted - now, we had to act faster than in the preceding months.

I relied on the medical expertise of physicians from the university hospital and on March 8, 2004 began to take the first pills as part of my hormone therapy.

That started the triple therapy suggested by urologists in cooperation with the experts on medical radiology and radiotherapy, comprising:

- Hormone therapy,
- Radical brachytherapy and
- Radiotherapy of lymph drainage areas...

A Warning from the Hospital

Three days after the start of the treatment, a letter arrived from the university hospital. I was informed that for this "treatment option", that is, for the described combination of therapies, there was "no secure scientific data", and I was warned of the possible consequences.

Only now it became clear to me that in conventional oncology there was no reliable and promising approach for my case.

Furthermore, I was informed that in case of the proposed therapy failing again (which would only become clear in two years), conventional medicine would no longer be able to help me!

And I Would Be Considered "Incurably Ill"!

After lengthy discussions with my dear wife, I immediately terminated the hormone therapy that I already started, that is, I stopped taking the preparation and "forgot to buy a syringe in the pharmacy".
I did not want to be a guinea pig!

My Salvation: the Breuss Cancer Treatment!

So, two and a half long years had passed since I was diagnosed with cancer. I did not know what to do.

Chapter 2 - How I Conquered Cancer in 42 Days ...

In any case, I did not in the least want to go through triple therapy.

Quite by chance I learned, from a business partner of mine, about a man who belonged to his customers and who five years ago had
"starved his cancer to death".
For me, it was a totally unbelievable story which I, of course, started to pursue at once.

The former cancer patient, whose name was Edwin Schatz, not only confirmed his recovery, but also gave me a tip to find a small booklet by Rudolf Breuss, so that I was able to start my own fight against cancer.

According to him, I could be 100% sure that in 42 days time the cancer would be defeated.

I immediately bought Breuss' book "Natural Treatment of Cancer, Leukemia and Other Seemingly Incurable Diseases" and

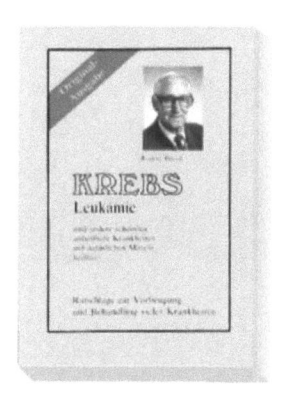

From March 15 to April 25, 2004

I underwent Breuss Cancer Treatment.

Chapter 2 - How I Conquered Cancer in 42 Days ...

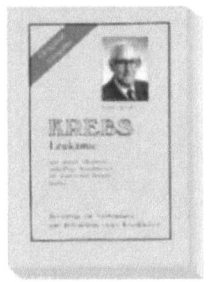

Rudolf Breuss
"Natural Treatment of **CANCER, LEUKEMIA,** AND OTHER SEEMINGLY INCURABLE DISEASES". GUIDE TO PREVENTING AND TREATING MANY DISEASES.
This book, which has sold over one million copies worldwide, represents the unmodified original edition, expanded and edited by Rudolf Breuss in 1990.
Published by the "Rudolf Breuss" private publishing house
A6, 164 pages, paperback,
€ (Germany) 10,70
ISBN 3-00-018407-4

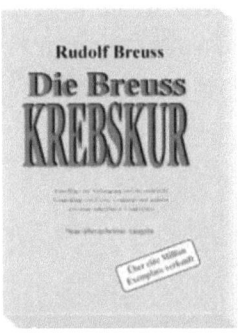

Rudolf Breuss
"The Breuss CANCER CURE"
Advice on Prevention and Natural treatment of Cancer, Leukemia and Other Seemingly Incurable Diseases.
Published by the "Rudolf Breuss" private publishing house
Updated edition – 2005
The bestseller of Rudolf Breuss now in a larger, practical format (A5).
Adapted by the publisher to the modern context.
A5, 120 pages, paperback,
€ (Austria, Switzerland) 13,90
ISBN 3-200-00429-0

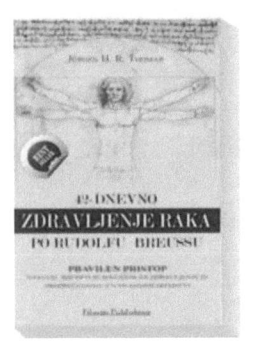

Jurgen H.R. Thomar
"Rudolf Breuss 42-day Cancer Treatment"
Filargo Publishing, 2011
250 p., 2011
Price 24,95 €
ISDN 978-9619-304518
This is the Slovenian edition of my book on cancer treatment.

Chapter 2 - How I Conquered Cancer in 42 Days ...

How I survived it:

My Treatment Diary

Three Days before the Treatment

I have thoroughly studied Breuss' book. While reading, I came to the conclusion that its content is poorly structured. You find **important tips** *here and there, then, some pages later, there is another chunk of important* **information** *however, they are often hidden in subordinate clauses or testimonials.*

Therefore, I work my way through the book twice, making notes and first of all trying to put things orderly and proper sequences in this "literary chaos". It is important to realize that Rudolf Breuss wrote his book late in his life and, unfortunately, got no assistance with editing the text.

In parallel with that, I experiment with making the Breuss juice using the available juice extractor. The first model is of no use and is replaced.

I also prepare the "shopping list". At the top of the list I indicate things that might not be available locally, for example, various herbal teas. I go to the city and inquire where to buy organic vegetables.

For me, a pre-made juice is out of the question. I want to follow Breuss' recommendation and make fresh juices at home.

In such a way I should be able to focus on the treatment and, by pressing juice and making herbal teas (I want to do everything myself!) to constantly renew my motivation.

So, three days slipped by and the evening before my treatment arrived.

Right before the Treatment

Do I have everything in place? All herbal teas? A precise kitchen scale and – for special teas where each 1, 2 or 3 grams are important – a letter weighing scale? Cups and pots for various teas?

Are my teapots and cardboards accurately labelled? Are there enough vegetables? Are the enough containers for the vegetable juices and prepared? Have I got a reliable juice extractor? Hawthorn drops? Onion? Vegetable bouillon cubes?

My dear wife "is allowed" only to clean the juice extractor, otherwise I would shove it completely into the dishwasher. Her competent hands will also handle the preparation of my "opulent" lunch. Everything else should be my job.

> **Tip:** *whenever possible, try to do everything related to your treatment by yourself. First of all, it is distracting, and, secondly, you come to sort of identify yourself with the treatment. I consider this to be very important.*

Have I taken precautions for an emergency: lemon juice? Sauerkraut juice? Savoy cabbage for a cabbage leaf compress? The last question is purely hypothetical since I decided not to make compresses. As to the tip regarding lemon juice and sauerkraut juice, I found it in Breuss' book only after finishing the treatment! ☺

The First Three Days

Everything is new to me: brewing teas in the volume prescribed and store for the whole day; lack of breakfast, the unusual "lunch" and again the absence of dinner.

Right from the outset, my wife and I were in agreement: I do the treatment, and she wholly supports me in it. For practical purposes, I relocated my meals – with the exception of "lunch" – to the kitchen. After all, here are my teas, tinctures, broths, as well as freshly pressed vegetable juice. And whenever I am near the kitchen, I take a sip.

Thus, my wife and I have hardly any contact with each other at breakfast and also at dinner: my wife eats as usual, at the dining table in the dining room, and I eat mainly in the kitchen.

The situation is completely different at lunch: my wife cooks for herself the dishes she likes. Every now and then, she likes to eat something special, which I normally don't get. It does not bother me, and I can easily watch her enjoying her food. Well, I have my "French onion soup" à la Breuss!

Three and a half kilometres of Nordic walking a day along wonderful forest paths in the surroundings help me to keep fit and distracted. Fortunately, the weather is favourable, so I can do sports despite the cold.

My biggest surprise is that I do not feel hungry! But I need to get used to, after the initial shock, the dark red stool (because of the beetroot!).

The Third Evening

My blood pressure stabilized at the ideal value of 125/75, notwithstanding my refusal of antihypertensive medication which I had taken for years. A pleasant surprise for me!

I also make the decision to discontinue my thyroid medication (as will be seen later, with surprising results), because Rudolf Breuss advises, as far as possible, against taking any medications during his treatment.

I am also aware that such refusal of medication must be properly considered in each individual case, with regard to the possible risks; in any case, it should be discussed with a physician.

At the beginning of the treatment my weight was an impressive 105 kg. By the evening of the third day I lost three kilograms, which did not hurt me at all. Also, according to the special body fat scale, my body fat values dropped by a whole three units – excellent! These are the results of physical activity.

Week One Is Over

I feel very well. As usual during therapeutic fasting, my body probably releases plenty of endorphins (see "Happiness hormones" in Chapter 6). I find daily sport activities quite distracting; moreover, I am planning to make a herb spiral in the garden. You have to do something. The information on this spiral is obtained from the Internet.

> **Tip:** *search, for example, Google, for a "herb spiral" if you also want to plant your herbs in the shape of a spiral, in order to make your lifestyle even healthier.* ☺

Weight loss in week one is 4.5 kg. After a week without solid food I felt better than I ever thought I would be. I have no difficulty in working at the PC. I have full concentration and can easily combine two things: working for the company and treatment for health. It is **important** *for me: a small software company should not suffer from the fact that its director is fasting.*

Even my leisure does not suffer from treatment. Mondays and Thursdays I meet my friends in a café – it's our fixed routine. I bring my special tea mix in a thermos bottle and ask the waiter to serve it as an inconspicuous wine spritzer (cold tea has the same colour). Of course, for a reasonable tip. ☺

Week Two

It is nice to do everything on my own: the teas and vegetable juice. It is distracting. And I tend to think that the quality of life is created by me! Only the "amazing" lunch - the culinary highlight of the day – is cooked by my dear wife.
Do I feel hungry? NOT at all. Sports: YES! Weight loss? Yes, already 8.5 kg!

Week Three

My cancer treatment has, in the meantime, become quite a routine. All treatment-related questions and problems are resolved in a much more casual way than at the beginning of the treatment.

My herb spiral is taking shape: I have removed the upper layer of soil (30 cm thick) on the plot with a diameter of 3 m; now it should be filled with a drainage layer of 30 cm.

In the meantime, it's April, which means warmer weather. But I notice that I get cold more than I am accustomed to at these temperatures.

My weight loss since the beginning of treatment is 14 kg.

Week Four

A "full" working week in the garden. The weather plays along, and I can "warm up" while working. The PC and the office must wait.

The lovely weather should be made full use of!

I feel perfectly well.

I can easily carry out even heavy manual work in the garden. Despite all the drudgery in the garden, my recreational sport is not cancelled: every day I do 3.5 km of Nordic walking through the forest. Happily so.

The herb spiral is growing upwards – notably, in the shape of a spiral. Hunger? Not in the slightest. It is hard to believe.

Lost another 3.5 kg. Perhaps it is because of the sports and hard manual work? I am not sorry about that since I am now approaching my ideal "fighting weight" of 85 kg (my height is 187 cm).

Week Five

The freedom of movement, including movement outside the home which I try to maintain, has justified itself (see Chapter 6). I can go anywhere, attend various events and, as far as possible, participate in social life.

But when planning, make sure you don't leave anything out:

We went to an evening musical event in a neighbouring village. As I thought the assembly hall would be arranged as for a lecture or a conference, I left my thermos bottle(s) at home. A mistake. Everywhere were tables and chairs and the visitors started to order large portions of food and to devour it publicly. Various drinks were passed here and there through the room... Only I had nothing. Not even water since I was not allowed to drink water. Though it was a difficult evening for me, I survived it.

My herb spiral is slowly approaching completion. One can already see what it will look like.

And the weight?

Now it goes several hundred grams up and then down, within a range of 2 kilograms.

It's gotten very cold – at least, I feel cold. However, a glance at the thermometer reveals that in reality it has not got colder. I get cold faster perhaps because now I lack "fat" for burning.

It is a new feeling for me, since I used to have warm hands; I used to...

Day 35

From now on, everything seems to be out of control... I am really sick of it all. Always the same teas and the vegetable juice which gets no better (at the beginning it tasted delicious!), no variety... I want to stop it, that's enough...

> ***Tip:*** *in December 2005, having gone through the treatment for the second time – this time purely for studying – I came to the conclusion that vegetable juice can be very tasty. Read more in Chapter 8.*

My dear wife intervenes: she motivates me to go on. She "begs" me to continue the treatment and not interrupt it one week before the end. She succeeds. I carry on.

> ***Tip:*** *since the time around day 35 is so dangerous for staying the course, I provide a special Appendix with particular tips dedicated to this period.*

The Last Week

Week six: my mood has improved, the critical point has passed. Soon all of this will be over: my herb spiral, as well as my cancer treatment.

One minor incident shows how seriously my wife and I take everything relating to the forbidden food and how dangerous, even fatal a thoughtless

Chapter 2 - How I Conquered Cancer in 42 Days ...

bite can be (an example can be found in the Appendix, "Day 35"). When planting the herb spiral, I filled it with plants from my garden, including chives. I took one plant and was a little uncertain whether it was really chives, for it was almost twice as high as a normal one. I broke its stem and was about to taste it. "Stop!" shouted my wife. "You may not eat anything!" And the stem flew in a high arc back to the garden-bed.
My weight is stabilized at 85 kg, which means my overall weight loss is 20 kg. My theoretical ideal weight is achieved! ☺

Breuss says his treatment results in weight loss of 5 to 15 kg. In my case, it was 20 kg. Perhaps, because of various tasks I kept myself busy with. And due to daily sports activities. And also because I was happy to loose these kilograms!

The First Days after the Treatment

At midnight on day 42, accurately to the second, i.e. immediately after the end of the course of treatment, I delight myself by slowly eating a banana. I never suspected bananas can taste so delicious!

> *Tip: during this period, one should probably be more careful. For example, start with some spoonfuls of vegetable soup with potatoes and carrots. It is also a good idea to eat a stale roll chewing it thoroughly – it readjusts your digestive system back to solid food. Read more about this in Chapter 6 "Fast breaking and readaptation".*

In the coming days and weeks I take only light food in small portions, i.e., I eat mainly vegetables and fish (instead of sausages and meat as I used to).

From the second week I allow myself larger portions. However, now I eat less than before the treatment.

Chapter 2 - How I Conquered Cancer in 42 Days ...

Thanks to this careful transition to eating, it causes no difficulties whatsoever, and food tastes as good as never before!

--------- **The Treatment Diary Ends Here.**

My Conclusion at the End of the Cancer Treatment

Reading the Breuss' booklet and conducting detailed studies of the theory of "starving the cancer" led me to developing a highly positive attitude to the treatment.

Careful preparation of all utensils, herbal teas, broths and tinctures made my transition from a "normal life" to the "Breuss-treatment phase" easy.

The cancer treatment – at least during its first four or five weeks – turned out easier to go through than I expected. And up to the time around day 35, I felt quite good.

My personal conviction is that it is indispensable to follow all the treatment procedures to the letter! Any deviation from, or modification of Breuss' recommendations, will cast doubt on the success of the treatment!

In difficult situations, I motivated myself by reading numerous testimonials in Breuss' book. So I believe that being a powerful motivator, the book is essential for the treatment.

It is noteworthy that through physical activity when walking and erecting the herb spiral, I lost weight but not muscle mass.

Switching to other activities is also **very important** – be it your job or hobby.

Weight loss should not be a cause for concern – the lost kilograms are regained (if you wish) very quickly!

The support of my dear wife was **immensely important** to me.

With her help I managed to cope with the hardships of the treatment and, specifically, overcome the crisis on and around day 35 – I am grateful to her with all my heart.

Chapter 2 - How I Conquered Cancer in 42 Days ...

Cancer Overcome with the Breuss Method

Two weeks after the treatment I visited an urologist (I had not consulted this specialist for a long time) to find out whether the cancer was actually overcome and how things might develop. At first the physician was extremely skeptical; he said it didn't matter whether I did the fasting therapy or not: cancer could not disappear just out of the blue!
However, when the laboratory test became known, when discussing them he said:
   "Mr. Thomar, something has happened to you!"

And I replied spontaneously: "Yes, I know – the cancer is gone!"

The PSA level turned out to be only 0.53 ng/ml of free PSA. It is equal to the normal value for a healthy man under 50. Now the urologist became much more interested and began to ask questions about my cancer history and the treatment which had just ended. He said that in four weeks there would be another examination and if the PSA level did not go up, I would be able to assume that the cancer had been overcome[3].

Further control examinations confirmed that my condition did not deteriorate; my PSA-levels, if listed in chronological order from May 21, 2004 to the summer of 2005, were as follows: 0.59 – 0.55 – 0.36 – 0.32 – 0.42 – 0.30. After the repeat cancer treatment that I went through in the autumn of 2005 for reasons of elaborating the Breuss Method, my PSA level was – believe it or not – 0.17, i.e. lower than ever.

---

[3] 4 days prior to every measurement of the PSA level, you should avoid cycling and sex, otherwise the values will not be correct!
Source: The Federal Association for Prostate Cancer Self-Help and Cancer Compass, Volker Karl Oehlrich Society.

Also read p. 121 "After treatment: taking control of success" and below

Chapter 2 - How I Conquered Cancer in 42 Days ...

On November 9, 2006 I asked my family doctor to check all major cancer markers. According to the laboratory report, all 16 values were within normal range.

The PSA levels, the **most important** tumour markers in my case, were as follows:

- PSA: 0.18 ng/ml (normal value: <4.00),
- Free PSA: 0.03 ng/ml,
- Complexed PSA: 0.15 ng/ml (normal value: <2.6),
- fPSA/ PSA-quotient 16.7 % (normal value> 18.00)

Overall judgment: PSA-level is normal.

During the next outpatient general preventive check-up conducted on 21.5.2007, the PSA tumor marker was measured at 0.28 ng/ml. In 2008, I did not measure this marker at all. As long as it remains below 4.0 ng/ml, I am absolutely happy. Also the current values from 2009 – 1.0 ng/ml – are completely normal, which fosters my belief in the healing effect of the Breuss Treatment.

The outpatient general preventive check-up conducted on 9.6.2009 in the city of Ulm, produced the following values:

- CEA tumor marker: 0.6 ng/ml
- PSA in the lower normal range: 0.69 ng/ml

In 2010, its value was again below 1.0. And on 30.8.2011 the free PSA value constituted 0.33 ng/ml. Thus, in the last nine years my PSA level has varied, with small swings, well below the normal value of 4.0 ng/ml. The arithmetic average of the measured values was exactly 0.43 ng/ml, that is, a normal value for a healthy **man under 50 years.**

Chapter 2 - How I Conquered Cancer in 42 Days ...

I am going on 75, what else can you ask for?

Therefore, I am going to control my PSA level once a year at the very most, as I feel cured!

> **The Cancer is gone!
> I have overcome it!**
>
> **Thank you, Rudolf Breuss!**

Due to the Breuss Cancer Treatment, My Thyroid Has Been Healed!

In the context of an aftercare examination in a military hospital four weeks after the end of the treatment, I also had my thyroid gland examined, since for some 40 years I had had an **under**active thyroid gland (hypothyroidism) and was on regular medication.

The results of the radioisotope examination were sensational: **under**activity was now replaced by latent **hyper**activity (hyperthyroidism).

However, this result had to be checked once again four weeks later, by means of nuclear medicine. Since we have the necessary equipment at the Pfullendorf hospital, four weeks later I went to the hospital and asked its chief physician, a good acquaintance of mine, to conduct this examination. Surprised, he asked me why.

I told him, *"Doctor B., I am asking you to examine my thyroid gland as a few weeks ago I finished my anti-cancer fasting therapy and it has cured me of cancer."* To which he responded, *"Oh, Mr. Thomar, no fasting therapy can possibly cure cancer!"*

Chapter 2 - How I Conquered Cancer in 42 Days ...

Three days after the examination I received a written report and tried to understand its contents, but I failed. Therefore, I called Doctor B. and asked him to "translate" the report for me (i.e., from medical jargon into comprehensible German).

I received the following answer: *"Mr. Thomar, two short sentences:*

- *Firstly: your thyroid is absolutely healthy!*
- *Secondly: we have screened you for cancer using major cancer markers.*

Mr. Thomar, congratulations!"

What else could you wish for? Two good pieces of news at once.

Thank you, Rudolf Breuss!

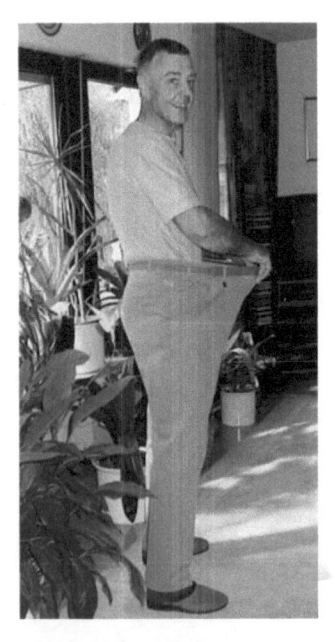

I no longer take thyroid medications; I only take iodine tablets which offset the iodine deficiency in southern Germany.

Weight Loss: Unavoidable Whilst Fasting

He who does not eat anything for 42 days, usually loses weight. Here I'm not actually telling you anything new. It is not always so, but with me it was just the case. Being 187 cm tall, my body weight during the treatment was reduced from 105 kg by 20 kg and reached 85 kg.

Chapter 2 - How I Conquered Cancer in 42 Days ...

The trousers shown in the photo were bought shortly before the treatment, when I did not yet know that I would be soon going through the Breuss Cancer Treatment.

I could advertise slimming products with this photo. Here's the dynamics of my weight loss:

- After one week: by 4,5 kg
- After two weeks: by 8,5 kg
- After three weeks: by 14,0 kg
- After four weeks: by 17,5 kg
- After six weeks: by 20,0 kg

Keep in mind that during the treatment I did physical exercises and worked in the garden constructing a herb spiral.

Rudolf Breuss writes that patients do not lose much weight during his cancer treatment. However, one may expect to lose from 5 to 15 kg (based on the patient's initial weight and his engagement in physical work and active sports during the treatment). Breuss' book mentions that those patients who have lost a lot of weight prior to the cancer treatment (for example, losing 10 kg from the initial 55 kg before the treatment), can also successfully go through the treatment.

As I have learned in many conversations and experienced during several fasting rounds I have undertaken, and as can be seen from the Oncological report, patients usually regain their normal body weight within four weeks after the treatment (see the Oncological report). An extract from it is provided in Chapter 12; for the original report see Bibliography.

Of course, it is possible to stabilize the attained and desired weight loss by means of a change in eating habits and physical activity. Personally I, within the first four weeks after the treatment, again gained nine kilograms and reached the weight which I would like to retain. This has come to nothing, however: I have again returned to the weight I had before the treatment. ☺

How Long Can a Human Fast?

For 48 days I drank nothing but pure water

People sometimes demonstrate amazing things in terms of persistence. On page 27, I already told you the story of a female doctor who in the early 1980s fell ill with cancer. She had not yet heard about Breuss, however, she knew about the remedial powers of fasting. So, for 48 (!) days she went without eating and drank nothing but pure water. The lady lost a lot of weight and reached an incredible 25 kg. At that time she was pregnant and during the fasting period gave birth to a baby. The baby girl was born healthy and developed quite adequately; she is about 30 years old now. Mrs. P., Dr. Med., upon completion of her fast was healed of cancer, and so far the disease has never returned.

Thus, fasting over a long period can be very effective. However, the Breuss fasting treatment is not so strict, and it is not so difficult to get through, since over all 42 days patients receive a whole range of essential foods and drinks.

80 Days without Food Are Probably the Maximum

The newspaper report with the headline "The Maximum Lies at 80 Days", which addressed the hunger strike of Yulia Tymoshenko, renewed my interest in this. The author of the article, therapist Sigrun Merger, associate professor and an expert on internal medicine with specialization in endocrinology (study of hormones), diabetes and metabolism at the University Hospital of Ulm, shares her experiences with respect to fasting.

Chapter 2 - How I Conquered Cancer in 42 Days ...

The human body has, since the Stone Age, been geared for long periods of starvation. It is known from literature that a person of normal weight can survive without food for some 60 days. The maximum is 80 days. However, it depends on the muscle and fat mass of the body. Besides, within a period of eight to ten days, the metabolism is reduced by around 50%.

Science Discovers the Hunger Cure

It has long been known that short-term fasting may have a useful impact on treating various diseases. Take rheumatism, high blood pressure, migraine or allergies – abstaining from food over a limited period of time mostly combined with subsequent change in diet helped many patients, says Dr. Francoise Wilhelmi de Toledo. She runs the Buchinger therapeutic fasting clinic on Lake Constance together with her husband.

Now, a report arrives from North America which establishes a link between fasting and cancer therapy: the biologist and gerontologist Valter Longo, professor at the University of Southern California in Los Angeles succeeded in improving, through fixed-term fasting, the effectiveness of chemotherapy in mice with cancer. His research results were published in February 2012 in the professional journal "Science Translational Medicine".

Longo treated mice with cytostatics (substances impeding cell growth, a drug against autoimmune diseases, substances that inhibit the cell division process), whereby one group had previously been exposed to hunger, and another group was not.

The group exposed to hunger survived, while mice in the other group did not.

This was the starting point for another research series which is currently (2012/2013) running and attracting considerable attention. Initial tests with patients appear to be very promising. However, fasting prior to the administration of cytostatics lasts for only two days. Oncologists believe that due to this, the dosage of cytostatics can be increased, but they don't consider the question as to whether fasting alone could produce the effect.

Another experimental object Longo has been studying for years, is a common yeast strain found on the outer skin of Californian grapes. Yeast cells are easy to handle under laboratory conditions, and they can easily tolerate a switch from favorable to unfavorable nutritional conditions. Valter Longo and his team found that the yeast cells which were swimming in an aqueous solution without nutrients show better results in withstanding the attack of so-called oxidative stress than their "family members" living in a sugar solution. Oxidative stress is taken to mean, for example, free radicals or other chemical substances which damage the DNA and which can eventually cause cells to die. In further experiments, he substituted normal yeast cells with those with cancer genes and came to different results: under fasting conditions such cancerous yeast cells were more sensitive to damaging substances than well-nourished cancer cells.

"Fasting seems to protect only healthy cells", Longo says, summarizing his findings

Source: www.gesundheit.com / MediaDomain Verlags GmbH

Chapter 3

Cancer Treatment

⌘

Surgery without a Scalpel

Rudolf Breuss also calls his cancer cure "surgery without a scalpel".

As a healer, he considers cancer to be an autonomous tumor which grows slowly in the beginning, then grows faster and faster, making its transition into a cancerous tumor.

Breuss says that cancer lives mainly on protein, extracting it from solid food. But if the body is deprived of solid food, the protein-starved blood cells absorb everything nonessential, such as growths, waste matters, boils and tumors including those of a cancerous nature.

According to Breuss, blood flows to each and every spot of the body and produces a systemic impact on them. This is also true of metastases, which cannot be eliminated by performing a traditional operation – they are washed by blood and 'dried' in the way described above.

Thus, the Breuss Cancer Cure acts in the most accurate way, just like an operation, but without using a scalpel.

At the same time, the best possible combination of vegetable juice and recommended teas, broths and tinctures provides the patient's body with vitally important vitamins, minerals and trace elements.

Chapter 3 - Cancer Treatment

Treatment Directions

For cancer prevention and treatment, please follow the directions below:

- No food whatsoever for 42 days,
- Take only the vegetable juices recommended,
- Take only the herbal teas recommended,
- For lunch, have nothing but the items prescribed, and
- Take small doses of hawthorn tincture to improve heart function.

Though this method of cancer treatment is sometimes also called *"juice treatment"*, it mainly consists of these four elements.

During the treatment, it is better to drink freshly pressed juices if you have access to fresh, organic vegetables.

If such vegetables are not accessible then, according to Breuss, you should use a ready-made organic "Breuss Vegetable Juice Mix" (see Chapters 8 and 11).

Your approximate daily routine which, undoubtedly, may and must be adapted to your own needs, can be found on the following pages, as well as in the Appendix where it is designed as a chart.

Please note: Rudolf Breuss stresses that:

> *The treatment can only fail when my instructions are not strictly observed in all aspects*

Chapter 3 - Cancer Treatment

Daily Breuss Treatment Plan ...

Herbal teas and vegetable juices can be prepared early in the morning or the night before. It depends on individual peculiarities of the person who undertakes the task of preparing them. But it's preferable for the patients to prepare everything themselves in order to virtually 'live' their therapy.

If you decide to prepare herbal teas and juice in the morning, your daily routine may be as follows:

Early morning

• First on an empty stomach slowly drink one half cup of cold kidney tea.

• To support the heart function, take, depending on your body size, 20-40 drops of hawthorn tincture.

• Then comes the time to make herbal teas, which are taken warm.

• In 30 to 60 minutes after the kidney tea, take 1-2 cups of warm sage tea with St. John's wort, peppermint and balm, which are the components of the "Breuss Original Sage Tea" mixture.

• Now it's time to press vegetable juice. If you drink a ready-made juice, this step, of course, is skipped. ☺

• 30 to 60 minutes later, take a *small mouthful* of vegetable juice, and do not swallow it right away, but keep the juice in your mouth for a few moments!

• 15 to 30 minutes later, take another small mouthful of

Chapter 3 - Cancer Treatment

vegetable juice, depending on how hungry you are.

In the morning

- In the morning vegetable juice is to be taken approximately 10 to 15 times. Drink it only when you want it. But remember: juice is your nutrition now!

- In this way, drink at least 1/16 liter of vegetable juice, that is, half a coffee cup, and at most 1/4 liter of juice during the whole morning.

- In between drink sage tea made from the Breuss original sage tea mixture, which can now be taken cold and in any desired quantity.

- But: you **never add sugar** to any herbal teas during the treatment period!

From morning till noon

- This is a time period lasting 4 to 5 hours, during which you can do your work or pursue other activities such as sports.

At noon

- Slowly drink another one half cup of cold kidney tea.

- Your "lunch" includes 1 to 2 bowls of onion broth or only in case of liver or gall bladder problems, the broth is substituted with tea made from bean pods.

In the afternoon

- You will frequently need small mouthfuls of vegetable juice. No more than half a liter, but <u>at least</u> 1/8 liter of juice can be taken per day.

Chapter 3 - Cancer Treatment

From noon till evening

- Once again, you have a time period of 4 to 5 hours to attend to your work and other matters or go in for sports.

In the evening

- Before going to sleep drink another one half cup of cold kidney tea (but only during the first three weeks of treatment).

- In the evening there must be one half cup of kidney tea left. Keep it, for it'll have to be taken cold again next morning.

Throughout the day

- You also need to take a cup of cold cranesbill tea (herb Robert), sipping it by the mouthful, as well as a cup of warm or cold marigold tea. Each time you are in the kitchen or close to a place where you keep teas, you can have a mouthful or two.

- Drink at least one cup of a special herbal tea mix; it can be taken in any desired quantity.

- Depending on the cancer type, take special herbal teas (Chapter 10).

- In between vegetable juice and tea intakes, it is advisable to have an interval of 5 to 10 minutes.

- Throughout the day, cancer patients are recommended to have cabbage compresses (Chapter 4 – "Special Compresses – Cabbage Leaf Compress". These compresses are a must only for those with liver cancer, for all other cases they are an optional recommendation).

Chapter 3 - Cancer Treatment

Additional teas for various types of cancer

- Eye Cancer: one cup of cold eyebright tea per day, swallowed slowly.

- Breast, Ovarian and Uterine Cancers: drink one cup of cold tea made from lady's mantle or silvery lady's mantle together with a pinch of white or yellow dead nettle per day. Swallow slowly.

- Cerebral Tumor: swallow slowly one to two cups of cold balm mint tea per day.

- Stomach Cancer: swallow slowly one cup of cold wormwood tea or centaury tea per day.

- Prostate and Testicular Cancers: throughout the day, sip two cups of cold willow herb tea.

- Gall Bladder Cancer: swallow slowly one cup of *warm* or *cold* wormwood tea per day.

- Liver Cancer: swallow slowly two cups of *warm* or *cold* potatoes' skin tea per day. Additionally, apply cabbage leaf compresses.

- Spleen and Pancreatic Cancers: drink at least 1 liter of warm or cold sage tea made from the Breuss original sage tea mixture per day.

- Cancer of the Palate, Lips, Tongue, Lymph Nodes and Larynx: rinse your mouth and gargle with pimpernel tea (Pimpinella magna). There are special rules to be followed, see Chapters 4 and 10.

Chapter 3 - Cancer Treatment

- Skin Cancer: if the affected area is approximately ½ to 1 cm in diameter, swab it several times throughout the day with fresh greater celandine juice. There is a note to be followed, see Chapter 4!

Chapter 4

Differentiated Treatment for Various Types of Cancer

⌘

The scope of cancer treatment: from the eyes to the tongue

The treatment for all types of cancer is largely the same. However, some types require additional herbal teas, tinctures, certain ingredients as well as special procedures to be taken. Various tea recipes can be found below and in Chapter 10.

Eye cancer

This type of cancer is treated with vegetable juices and herbal teas alongside 42 days of abstinence from food.
Additionally you should have one cup of cold eyebright tea, swallowed slowly.
Preparation: steep a pinch of the herb in one cup of hot water for 10 minutes.

Pancreatic cancer

This cancer type is treated with vegetable juices and herbal teas alongside 42 days of abstinence from food.
Additionally, drink at least 1 liter of warm or cold sage tea made from the Breuss original sage tea mixture per day. Also recommended is a hot wrap made from grass flowers (Graminis flos), horsetail or oat straw. Prepare this wrap only if you know how to do wraps, otherwise it could do more

Chapter 4 - Differentiated Treatment for Various Types of Cancer

harm than good. A quick guide for wraps can be found in "Special wraps" at the end of this chapter.

Breast cancer

This type of cancer is treated with vegetable juices and herbal teas alongside 42 days of abstinence from food. Additionally, drink one cup of cold tea made from lady's mantle or silvery lady's mantle together with a pinch of white or yellow dead nettle per day, swallowed slowly.

Intestinal cancer

This type of cancer is treated with vegetable juices and herbal teas alongside 42 days of abstinence from food. I believe that there is no need to take any additional herbal teas or carry out special procedures for intestinal cancer, as Breuss' book says nothing about this.

Ovarian cancer

This form of cancer is treated with vegetable juices and herbal teas alongside 42 days of abstinence from food. Additionally, drink one cup of cold tea made from lady's mantle or silvery lady's mantle together with a pinch of white or yellow dead nettle per day, swallowed slowly.

Gall bladder cancer

This type of cancer is treated with vegetable juices and herbal teas alongside 42 days of abstinence from food. Additionally, drink one cup of cold tea made from lady's mantle or silvery lady's mantle together with a pinch of white or yellow dead nettle per day, swallowed slowly.

Chapter 4 - Differentiated Treatment for Various Types of Cancer

Preparation: in the first five or six days of treatment steep one small pinch of wormwood in a cup of hot water for 10 seconds. From the 7th day onwards, steep it for only 3 seconds not to make it too strong.

Note: with gall bladder cancer during your "lunch" never eat a whole bowl of onion broth in one sitting! It's better to take some 10 tablespoons of hot broth every hour.

Palate cancer

This type of cancer is treated with vegetable juices and herbal teas alongside 42 days of abstinence from food.
Additionally, gargle your mouth and throat with a tablespoon of pimpernel tea (Lat. Pimpinella), then spit it out. Do the same with the second tablespoonful. After gargling your mouth and throat with the third tablespoonful, swallow it. Do this several times per day.
Preparation: boil one teaspoonful of pimpernel herb in a full cup of water for 3 minutes several times per day.

Uterine cancer

This form of cancer is treated with vegetable juices and herbal teas alongside 42 days of abstinence from food.
Additionally, drink one cup of cold tea made from lady's mantle or silvery lady's mantle together with a pinch of white or yellow dead nettle per day, swallowed slowly.

Cerebral tumor

This form of cancer is treated with vegetable juices and herbal teas alongside 42 days of abstinence from food.
Additionally, slowly swallow one or two cups of cold balm

mint tea. For this, you can use Geminate horsemint or lemon balm mint, or mix them.

Cancer of the neck lymph nodes

This type of cancer is treated with vegetable juices and herbal teas alongside 42 days of abstinence from food.
Additionally, gargle your mouth and throat with a tablespoon of pimpernel tea (Lat. Pimpinella), then spit it out. Do the same with the second tablespoonful. After gargling your mouth and throat with the third tablespoonful, swallow it. Do this several times per day.
Preparation: boil one teaspoonful of pimpernel herb in a full cup of water for 3 minutes several times per day.

Skin cancer

This form of cancer is treated with vegetable juices and herbal teas alongside 42 days of abstinence from food.
Besides, if the affected area is approximately ½ to 1 cm in diameter, swab it several times throughout the day with fresh greater celandine juice (Chelidonium majus). Pluck the stem, squeeze its yellow bitter juice and apply to the affected area several times a day.
If the spot is larger, *apply the juice of greater celandine only to its edges touching the healthy skin.*
In winter use greater celandine herb tea for swabbing, but only around the affected area.
Preparation: put a pinch of greater celandine herb into a cup of hot water and let steep for 10 minutes. Apply still warm. Alternatively, use greater celandine tincture.
Note: never apply greater celandine juice, tea or tincture to open wounds!

Chapter 4 - Differentiated Treatment for Various Types of Cancer

Testicular cancer

This type of cancer is treated with vegetable juices and herbal teas alongside 42 days of abstinence from food.
Additionally, throughout the day, sip two cups of cold willow herb tea.

Cancer of the larynx

This form of cancer is treated with vegetable juices and herbal teas alongside 42 days of abstinence from food.
Additionally, gargle your mouth and throat with a tablespoon of pimpernel tea (Lat. Pimpinella), then spit it out. Do the same with the second tablespoonful. After gargling your mouth and throat with the third tablespoonful, swallow it. Do this several times per day.

Bone cancer

This type of cancer is treated with vegetable juices and herbal teas alongside 42 days of abstinence from food.
I believe that there is no need to take any additional herbal teas or carry out special procedures for bone cancer, as Breuss' book says nothing about it.

Liver cancer

This form of cancer is treated with vegetable juices and herbal teas alongside 42 days of abstinence from food.
In this case it is crucial to add raw potato juice to the freshly pressed vegetable juice. In case of raw potato intolerance, there exists an alternative option (see Chapter 8 "Special juice").
Additionally, slowly swallow one cup of cold wormwood tea per day.

Chapter 4 - Differentiated Treatment for Various Types of Cancer

Preparation: the first five or six days of treatment, steep one small pinch of wormwood in in a cup of hot water for 10 seconds. From the 7th day onwards, steep it for only 3 seconds, so as not to make it too strong.
Besides, slowly swallow two cups of warm or cold potatoes' skin tea per day.
Preparation and application: boil a handful of raw potato skins in two full cups of water for 2 to 4 minutes. If this tea tastes agreeable, then your liver needs it. If it tastes disagreeable, you do not need it.
If you suffer from liver cancer, it is necessary to prepare cabbage leaf compresses followed by rubbing with olive oil or St. John's wort oil (St. John's wort tea diluted with olive oil, 1:5 ratio). The instructions for preparing cabbage leaf compresses can be found in "Special compresses" at the end of this Chapter.

Note: during your "lunch" never eat a whole bowl of onion broth in one sitting! It's better to take some 10 tablespoons of hot broth every hour.

Leukemia

Leukemia is treated with vegetable juices and herbal teas, but without 42 days of abstinence from food.
In this case you need to drink ¼ liter of vegetable juice per day, keeping it in your mouth for some time and only then swallow it. Taking solid food is acceptable, but no meat soups, dishes made from beef or pork. Vegetable juice is sipped throughout the day, mainly before meals. In his book Breuss says, "The portal venous system surely absorbs the concentrated vitamins, as well as any other food." During the treatment period it is necessary to drink sage tea made from the Breuss original sage tea mixture, and for the first three

Chapter 4 - Differentiated Treatment for Various Types of Cancer

weeks kidney tea is to be taken as well.
Besides, in case of leukemia, just like in daily life in general, it is important not to have mouth poisons at home (Chapter 7). As a patient, I recommend you read pages 69 to 74 headlined "A simple way to treat leukemia by my method" of Breuss' original book.

Lip cancer

Lip cancer is treated with vegetable juices and herbal teas alongside 42 days of abstinence from food.
Additionally, gargle your mouth and throat with a tablespoon of pimpernel tea (Lat. Pimpinella), then spit it out. Do the same with the second tablespoonful. After gargling your mouth and throat with the third tablespoonful, swallow it. Do this several times per day.

Lung cancer

Lung cancer is treated with vegetable juices and herbal teas alongside 42 days of abstinence from food.
I believe that there is no need to take any additional herbal teas or carry out special procedures for lung cancer, as Breuss' book says nothing about this.

Lung tuberculosis

Tuberculosis, though not a form of cancer, can also be beaten with the Breuss therapy, in which case the disease is treated with vegetable juices and herbal teas alongside 42 days of abstinence from food.
Additionally, swallow one teaspoonful of broadleaf plantain seeds with some water or tea. In pharmacies broadleaf plantain seeds are sold as Indian plantago seeds.

Chapter 4 - Differentiated Treatment for Various Types of Cancer

Cancer of the lymph nodes

This form of cancer is treated with vegetable juices and herbal teas alongside 42 days of abstinence from food.
I believe that there is no need to take any additional herbal teas or carry out special procedures for this type of cancer, as Breuss' book says nothing about it.

Stomach cancer

This type of cancer is treated with vegetable juices and herbal teas alongside 42 days of abstinence from food.
Additionally, sip one cup of cold wormwood tea or centaury tea per day.
Preparation: steep a pinch of wormwood herb (Lat. Artemisa absinthium) or centaury herb (Lat. Centaurium erythraea) for 3 seconds in a cup of hot water.
Should the patient also suffer from irritable bowel syndrome, besides the treatment described above, he should take one more cup of valerian tea with wormwood (where wormwood is taken to mean the medicinal plant of Artemisa absinthium, and not an alcoholic beverage, though in German both words sound identical – Wermut).
Preparation: boil one half teaspoon of valerian root in a cup of water for 3 minutes, then add a pinch of wormwood and boil for another 3 seconds.
If the patient has vegetable juice intolerance and vomits frequently, he should take 3 drops of tormentil tea in the morning and in the evening. More details can be found on page 44 of the book "CANCER/leukemia".

Spleen cancer

This form of cancer is treated with vegetable juices and herbal teas alongside 42 days of abstinence from food.
Additionally, drink at least 1 liter of warm or cold sage tea made from the Breuss original sage tea mixture per day. Also recommended is a hot wrap, see page 83, made from grass flowers, horsetail or oat straw. The grass flowers are just left to steep, horsetail and oat straw are boiled for 10 minutes.

Disseminated sclerosis

Note: Disseminated sclerosis is not cancer. Nevertheless, on Breuss' advice, I list here his recommendations on how to treat this disease. Patients cured of pseudosclerosis by him had symptoms similar to those of real disseminated sclerosis. According to Breuss, in case of real disseminated sclerosis, one or several nerve fibers become cut, thus making this disease incurable.

Such disseminated sclerosis is treated with vegetable juices and herbal teas alongside 42 days of abstinence from food. In addition, breathing exercises are to be done as described on pages 106 to 107 in the "High blood pressure" chapter in the book "CANCER/leukemia". But in the case mentioned here, breathing exercises are to be done 20 to 30 times per day for 5 to 10 minutes.

Kidney cancer

This type of cancer is treated with vegetable juices and herbal teas alongside 42 days of abstinence from food.
I believe that there is no need to take any additional herbal teas or carry out special procedures for this form of cancer, as Breuss' book says nothing about it.

Chapter 4 - Differentiated Treatment for Various Types of Cancer

Prostate cancer

This form of cancer is treated with vegetable juices and herbal teas alongside 42 days of abstinence from food.
Additionally, sip two cups of cold willow herb tea throughout the day. Preparation: steep a pinch of willow herb (Lat. Herba Epilobii parvifloris concis) in two cups of hot water for 10 minutes.

Tongue cancer

This type of cancer is treated with vegetable juices and herbal teas alongside 42 days of abstinence from food.
Additionally, gargle your mouth and throat with a tablespoon of pimpernel tea (Lat. Pimpinella), then spit it out. Do the same with the second tablespoonful. After gargling your mouth and throat with the third tablespoonful, swallow it. Do this several times per day.

Treating other types of cancer

If you have a different type of cancer not mentioned above, you would probably ask yourself if the Breuss treatment can help in your case.
Breuss' answer is absolutely clear:

YES, IT CAN

In his opinion, cancer is an autonomous tumor which grows slowly in the beginning, then grows faster and faster making its transition into a cancerous tumor.
Then Breuss says that cancer lives on protein, which it extracts from solid food. But if the body is deprived of solid food, the protein-starved blood cells absorb everything nonessential, such as growths, waste matters, boils and tumors.

Chapter 4 - Differentiated Treatment for Various Types of Cancer

Following Breuss line of reasoning means supporting the idea that, in general, both the type of cancer and its location in the body don't matter. The only problem to be solved lies in selecting the proper additional herbal teas to be taken. To my mind, the herbal tea to be taken is the one recommended for treating the organ which is the closest to your cancer-affected organ. For example, for thyroid cancer, the patient should additionally have pimpernel tea which is recommended for cancer of the lymph nodes.

Unfortunately, we can no longer ask Breuss himself. He would undoubtedly give us the best advice. However, taking into account the fact that, according to the Breuss way of treatment, the location of cancer in the body does not matter, my understanding cannot be wrong.

Anyway, personally I see the attempt to apply the Breuss therapy to treating a type of cancer not mentioned in this Chapter, as fully justified

Special compresses

For various types of cancer, the treatment, in addition to herbal teas and vegetable juice, should – and for many types has to – also include special compresses (wraps).

Cabbage leaf compress

For the evening compress take three savoy cabbage leaves and wash them in warm water until there is no dirt left on the leaves. The outside leaves are the best. Then roll the leaves with a bottle or rolling pin until all the veins on the cabbage leaves are rolled flat.

For beginners: to make a compress, put a folded wool blanket (folded approximately 50 cm wide) on your bed, place a linen

Chapter 4 - Differentiated Treatment for Various Types of Cancer

cloth over top (approximately 25 to 30 cm wide), on top of this place another such cloth with the three cabbage leaves (two leaves next to each other and one on top of them). Put the inside sheet with the cabbage leaves on the patient's back or onto the affected area.

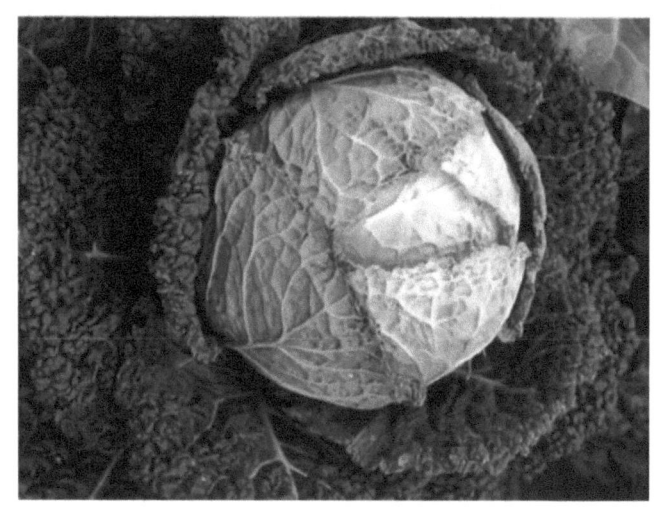

Savoy cabbage (Lat. Brassica oleracea)

After that fasten the linen cloth and then the blanket as tightly as possible. Such a compress shouldn't slip, sitting firmly in place, for it is left for the nighttime. If it hasn't been applied tightly, the patient will feel cold and the cabbage compress will have to be removed.

The following morning take off the compress, wash the area with warm water and dry off thoroughly with a towel. Then rub warm St. John's wort oil (one to two teaspoons of oil; St. John's wort steeped in olive oil at a ratio of 1:5; or ready-made oil bought in a pharmacy) onto the affected area and put a warm towel over it for a few minutes.

Before you undertake the cabbage leaf wrapping, the patient must get properly warm. He can stay in bed until his body is

warmed up, or go to bed which has been warmed up.
For more details concerning the above mentioned compresses, read the brochure "On the wonderful therapeutic effect of cabbage leaf", see Bibliography.

Hot wraps

This is the way of making a hot wrap of grass flowers, horsetail or oat straw (which can be bought at Dietary Products and Herbs Shops). Take a big enough linen cloth approximately 80 x 80 cm in size, fold it once and put aside. The folded cloth is to be bigger than the corresponding part of the patient's body. Dampen the cloth. For this put it into freshly boiled water, and after it is soaked through, squeeze it, having wrapped the cloth in the towel so as not to scald oneself.
The wearing of rubber gloves when squeezing is recommended so as not to scald oneself. Squeezing removes excess water. And the cloth is dampened to make it swollen.
Now put a handful of grass flowers, horsetail or oat straw on the side of the wet cloth which will be applied to the patient's body, fold it and place it carefully onto the affected area so that the patient doesn't get scalded.

When applying the compress, pay attention to the following:
1. No wrinkles on the cloth,

2. No empty space under the cloth, that's why it must be fastened tightly (but no occlusions, of course!)

3. All hot wraps must be applied quickly one after another (they may be folded first and then applied)

Then a suitable piece of flannel cloth or flannel towel is put on top (flannel is a good moisture absorber, it is fluffy and kind to the skin), tautened and fastened with safety pins. Finally,

Chapter 4 - Differentiated Treatment for Various Types of Cancer

the patient's entire body is covered with a bedspread up to the neck, or wrapped up in a woollen blanket.
Hot wraps are worn for about half an hour.
A hot wrap is to be removed before it gets cold.

〜〜
〜〜

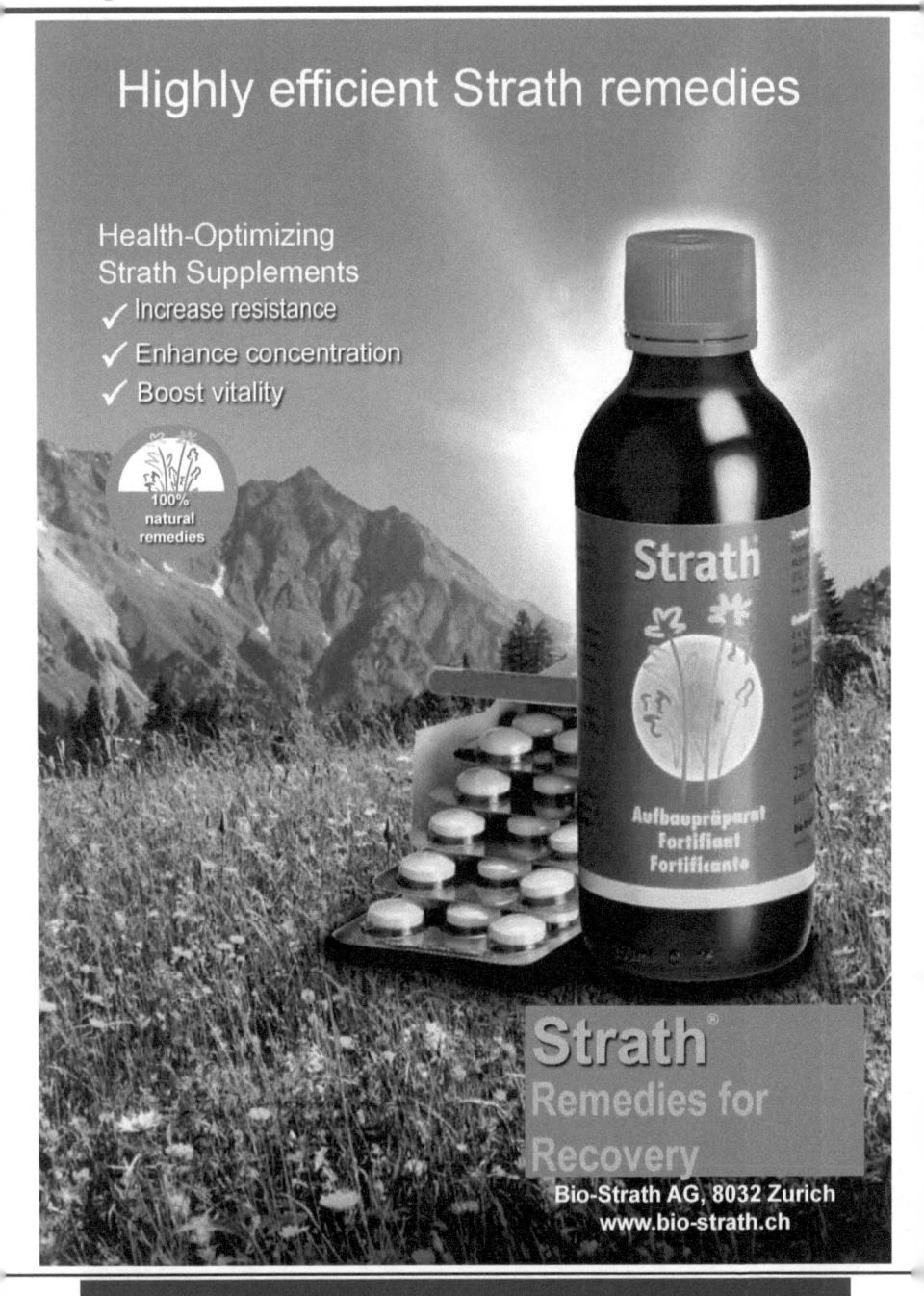

Chapter 4 - Differentiated Treatment for Various Types of Cancer

Highly efficient Strath remedies

Health-Optimizing Strath Supplements
- ✓ Increase resistance
- ✓ Enhance concentration
- ✓ Boost vitality

100% natural remedies

Strath
Aufbaupräparat
Fortifiant
Fortificante

Strath® Remedies for Recovery

Bio-Strath AG, 8032 Zurich
www.bio-strath.ch

Chapter 5
Searching for the Solution

⌘

Finding your own path

1. You obviously somehow got to know about the Breuss Total Cancer Treatment as you are reading these passages. Actually, it is not important how you got your hands on the book you're reading at the moment. Some people get their information on Breuss and his Total Cancer Treatment from their friends, families and acquaintances or through the Internet and other mass media. Other patients have found themselves in a life-threatening situation because conventional medicine failed to help them.

2. Dear Reader, what you're busy with right now is called extension of knowledge, which is absolutely the right thing to do, I should say. My book is aimed at helping you to get as much information on cancer and ways to treat it as possible. Unfortunately, your doctor didn't show you the path to naturopathy. Or perhaps he did?

3. Medical doctors are known to have different views on treatment itself. Some of them focus on the human being as a whole, and others put "pure" conventional medicine first. Others are indeed narrow-minded. And I'm going to prove it on the page below by demonstrating what can happen and what actually does happen to a patient after he is diagnosed with CANCER, and when, first of all, he has to come to terms with this terrible diagnosis. Unfortunately, without being given any time for that. All the necessary words of encouragement can be found on the page below:

Chapter 5 - Searching for the Solution

"You've got cancer..."

Take your time and never lose your head!

After all of a sudden you're diagnosed with cancer, your medical doctor (or doctors) can pressure you into making a hasty decision (you get the impression that you are deprived of the opportunity to ponder on the situation and gather any additional information), with their strict instructions and explicit intimidation, for example:

«I've made inquiries about a place in the cancer centre to be reserved for you, so you can be admitted to the hospital this week or next week at the latest. For <u>cancer</u>, every second count...» or

«You're having an operation next week. We've managed to find this opportunity for you», or

«You're starting your course of chemotherapy next week. Here is your appointment card for it...», or

«Such diagnosis gives us no time at all. The sooner you start the treatment, the better it is for you»...

<u>Try to keep calm,</u> thank your medical doctor and go home – <u>without making any arrangements to see them</u>. Tell them that you need to come to terms with this diagnosis and "digest" it.

What is really important for you now is to collect all the necessary information in a calm way. That is the information on the method of treatment most acceptable for you and whether the grounds for urgency and haste do really exist (in the majority of cases they don't!).

First and foremost, don't get intimidated!

These questions make your head spin:

- Is an operation really unavoidable? And what's more, an urgent one?
- Are there any other treatments in my case? Which ones?
- What's the hurry with this surgery?
- How harmful is chemotherapy?
- Is it true that 95% of patients who undergone chemotherapy die within the next 5 years? And only 2% survive?
- What critical and long-lasting harm will be caused to my immune system?
- What long-term effects should I take into account?
- Is there any other way out for me but an operation, hormone therapy, irradiation and chemotherapy? And what are my chances for recovery after all of that?
- Is there any chance at all of recovery?

Questions, questions, questions…

Someone draws your attention to the Breuss Total Cancer Treatment. You collect the information on the advantages of this natural method of treatment (this is what you're actually doing right now).

If you ask your medical doctor about the Breuss cancer treatment, the answers will be as follows:

«If you follow this treatment, you're gonna bite the dust in

Chapter 5 - Searching for the Solution

a week at the latest» (these quotes by medical doctors have been repeatedly communicated to me by many patients!), or «This treatment can do nothing but harm ...», or

«I must warn you: you're risking your life!», or

«Do not get fooled by this quackery!, or

«If you miss this particular term, I do not know if I'll be able to help you at all!»

What a horrible thing to hear! And these words are voiced by your medical doctor who has never heard of fasting therapy, has not been appropriately educated to be a professional in this field, and who knows that conventional medicine is able to cure only three out of ten cancer patients. The other seven are dismissed as "hopeless cases" who are just out of luck!

But let's keep searching for the solution:

Chapter 5 - Searching for the Solution

4. Let's move along your own path: first, check if your type of cancer is on the list of various cancer types mentioned in Chapter 4 that are successfully cured following the Breuss Total Cancer Treatment. If your type is not on the list, I still recommend following this treatment for the reasons given in "Treating other types of cancer" (Chapter 4).

5. If you consider the Breuss Cancer Treatment as a possible route in fighting cancer, reflect on whether you will be able to go through 42 days of fasting. You might be overweight, just like I was back in the day, so you would be able to get your needs met, wouldn't you?

6. If you're not overweight, you should weigh your chances of victory over the tumor against the supposed risk of temporary weight lost together with your medical doctor, if possible.

7. Elderly ladies and gentlemen may, when making the decision of choosing this or that cancer treatment, be motivated by the following quote from Breuss, «*I'd like to point out that elderly people find it easier to go through my treatment as they have a better tolerance to a fast and do not need as much fibre*». However, this statement is not supposed to put younger patients off. As a rule, they have "a larger factor of safety" than elderly people.

8. What is to be done if your medical doctor comes to the conclusion that the Breuss Total Cancer Treatment is not for you? In this case it is quite possible that your doctor doesn't believe in the healing power of a fast or fasting therapy, and even considers it to be dangerous. It is also possible that the doctor doesn't know much about fasting therapy or has never studied this treatment. Do not blame

Chapter 5 - Searching for the Solution

him for that – instead, go to another doctor, and preferably to a fasting therapist who will be able to adequately assess your chances of going through this treatment. All the necessary addresses can be found in the Appendix (Address Directory).

9. What should be done if the treatment undergone hasn't produced any results, or chemotherapy has made you so debilitated that you lack the strength to take up the Breuss Cancer Treatment with its rather high demands (such as no solid food, physical exercises and fresh air)? Rudolf Breuss provides hope even for the "hopeless", those cancer-stricken men and women abandoned by conventional medicine. He says: «*And many of those patients who got operated, irradiated or underwent chemotherapy still have a chance to be healed*». He describes a case of a woman who being 10 kilos underweight (45 kilos instead of 55) went through the course of treatment and recovered. Chapter 12 "Conventional Medicine Test for the Breuss Total Cancer Treatment" shows that even those patients who had only several weeks left to live followed the course of treatment successfully, that is, they overcame cancer.

10. Recommendations on the preparation of severely debilitated patients for this treatment are given in Chapter 6 "Are you too weak for the treatment?" However, even under such conditions, the main prerequisite for successful cancer treatment is as follows:

You must want it really badly!

11. Carefully choose the place for going through the course of treatment, either your home or a medical institution with specially trained personnel (addresses of such medical

institutions can be found in the Appendix). I'm sure there are other medical institutions which specialize in fasting therapy. But make sure they carry out fasting therapy adequately, without providing additional food.

12. Only by having faith in your own will and strength, will you be able to start your treatment and survive it. Read success stories published in the original book by Rudolf Breuss, the stories of people who fought cancer with the Breuss Total Cancer Treatment, and ask yourself if you want the same and whether you believe in your own stamina.

13. In the book "CANCER/leukemia", an 87-year old F.B., Doctor of Medicine from Berchtesgaden, says, «*I consider the advanced and adapted to modern living Breuss Total Cancer Treatment as an opportunity to help cancer patients if they have enough courage and strength to go through this treatment*». He adds, «*In combination with strong faith, it can work miracles*». I would also like to add: you should and have to believe in the success of your anti-cancer treatment and your own stamina from the very start. Otherwise, there is no sense in starting fasting therapy.

14. Ask yourself what real alternatives you have. Sometimes it is easier to passively follow all the procedures prescribed by conventional medicine, rather than take the initiative and responsibility for being healthy. When following the Breuss Cancer Treatment, you have a powerful ally on your side, and that is nature: you are healed by active elements of juice and herbal teas, as well as by your own immune system.

15. Can you imagine a situation when you make your decision in favor of the Breuss Treatment against the judgments of

Chapter 5 - Searching for the Solution

your friends or even your family members? Do you have anyone who is ready to move along this path with you, encouraging and supporting you all the time?

16. If you think that you have no time for going through such treatment, face the fact that you may very soon have ages of time at hand, but with no chance to change anything ...

17. If you've found answers to the questions given above, it is a moment to make your decision:

18. Let it be the decision in favor of treatment!

19. If you make a different decision, I urge you to read this book right to the end just for the fun of it.

20. But for those who choose treatment, reading the following chapters is a must.

CHAPTER 6
Important Tips on the Treatment

Before the Treatment

Read this book carefully and mark the statements applicable for your type of cancer. Choose the right moment for the beginning of treatment, if possible in two weeks or so.

However, before starting the treatment you should plan at least seven days of preparation. They will be a transition from hectic and strenuous everyday life to the more contemplative days of treatment. These days will help you to change your attitude from common consumption to conscious self-containment. During this week you should consult your doctor so as to decide whether or not your health allows fasting.

Medical Supervision

It would be desirable if your treatment were accompanied by a physician who is always available with help and advice. How could, or should, this support look like?

1. During the first medical examination an assessment should be made of whether your current physical condition allows the 42-day treatment.
2. Control of blood pressures before, during (approximately in the middle of the treatment) and 14 days after the treatment ensures that your blood pressures are in the "green range". Your doctor should be available during the treatment to answer any questions or to support activities as a competent partner.
3. After the treatment, the final examination (the results your doctor will discuss with you) should show its outcome.

Chapter 6 - Important Tips on the Treatment

As this takes place, further diagnostic and, possibly, therapeutic strategy can be planned jointly.

Regrettably, many physicians consider fasting in principle as harmful – possibly because they have not heard about it during their training. If also your doctor was from the same group, I would recommend that you find a fasting doctor who knows what benefit people may derive from fasting. You can find the relevant addresses in the appendices and, of course, in the Internet. Perhaps your doctor knows such a specialist. Ultimately, it is entirely up to you whether or not you conduct the treatment under the supervision of a doctor (family doctor?) and/or in cooperation with a medical practitioner (naturopath).

Breuss comments: *"As I said earlier, I have always suggested medical supervision during the Total Cancer Treatment. I have done that so that the doctors could observe with me the progress of the treatment and the patient's health. They could check the patient's blood pressure and if the blood pressure was too low, prescribe a heart medication. However, over the I found that many orthodox medical doctors do not believe in this type of natural healing or natural remedies and will try to talk their patients out of taking this juice treatment, and also administer drugs which is, combined with my juice treatment, absolutely not good."*.

I myself informed my family doctor 14 days <u>after</u> beginning the treatment that I was undergoing treatment. After a short examination I received the "green light" from him. For the protection and strengthening of my immune system he prescribed me selenium[*)].

In the fifth week of fasting I provided my family doctor an interim report about the progress of treatment and my condition. He joyfully acknowledged **the** good news about the success of the treatment and my diagnostic values, which were within the normal range. If he had reacted in a different way, I would have nevertheless continued with the treatment, as I was sure that it

Chapter 6 - Important Tips on the Treatment

was exactly the right decision for me.

Spiritual and Mental Preparation

You should not "stumble" into the Breuss Total Cancer Treatment but prepare yourself inwardly for fasting! The required recommendations you will find in the book "Cancer, Leukemia and Other Seemingly Incurable Diseases, But Curable through Natural Means" and also in this book.

Prepare yourself mentally not to eat anything in the course of subsequent days and weeks. It would also be useful if you would undertake all the necessary preparations for the cancer treatment *by yourself*, i.e. if you were to purchase herbal teas, vegetables, hawthorn drops, etc. by yourself wherever possible.

A few day prior to the treatment, just "switch off". Enjoy fresh air in beautiful surroundings spend more time in nature. Don't watch TV for a couple of days – you will not miss a lot of things.

Take time out and concentrate on the upcoming treatment – for this half a day is sufficient, or just half an hour.

Thoughts of an elderly fasting doctor from Berchtesgaden will be helpful for you, who cites on pages 33 and 34 of the original Breuss book the natural healer with: *"We must destroy the cancerous tumour by starving it with the juice fasting"*, and he continues: *"Those*

---

*) As an important trace element selenium is indispensable for people. In fact, this element carries out a wide variety of jobs in the human body. Thus, this element is of great importance e.g. for cell and energy metabolism, the thyroid gland and immune system. Experts particulary stress the role of selenium in protecting our health and as means for preventing various diseases. The reason: selenium has antioxidant properties and it protects, accordingly, our cells from the harmful actions of free radicals as well as from negative environmental effects.

Source: www.medizin.de

Chapter 6 - Important Tips on the Treatment

who know about fasting are aware of it since during fasting the body excretes everything that does not belong inside and, in fact, separates everything malignant from healthy as long as the body has sufficient reserves of energy and the patient retains a strong faith in his or her internal divine healing power. This last point is the most important".

This doctor adds: *"Anyone failing to notice the soul and spiritual aspect of fasting will not go far. We need to always be clear that faith is a universal healing principle, and that without it little will be achieved".*
Well, there is nothing to add in my mind.

Then say to yourself, loudly:

I have decided to fast for 42 days!
and
I want to beat the cancer with this treatment!

These two sentences will accompany you over the next six weeks – you will also support yourself by repeating them during the treatment as often as possible.
Complete your mental preparation with the scheduling of your intention. Decide on a period of 42 days in the near future. Start next week if possible!

Physical Preparation

Drink a Lot

The most important thing during the preparatory period: drink a lot. It should be at least 3 to 4 liters of liquids a day. Drink good water[4], herbal and fruit infusions, vegetable and

---

4) Good water – a foodstuff that was available here in Germany years ago. It is almost impossible to find "good water" today. And, if at all, only in a few springs in extensive woodland areas.
I have dedicated a special section in Chapter 7 to the issue of "good water" as well as to the issue of "good food"..

Chapter 6 - Important Tips on the Treatment

fruit juices, but not sweetened beverages!

It is also an advantage when you drink one or two weeks prior to the treatment, in addition to normal food, about a ¼ liter of vegetable juice a day to get used to it. Drink the juice slowly, in small sips, keeping it in the mouth to mix it well with saliva, before meals. On a practical level, you can drink the ready-made Breuss vegetable juice. If you do not like it just press your juice at home, as a preparation for the treatment.

You will have to say goodbye to coffee and cakes. Forget about stimulants such as alcohol and nicotine. You are not allowed to smoke during the treatment anyway. Why not quit right now? Your body will thank you for it.

Eat easily digestible foods

On the preparatory days you should eat very little. It would be best to eat easily digestible food which is low in fat and high in fibre (such as rice and potato dishes, steamed vegetables, fresh food, fruit and salads).

Please also refrain from sweets, tea, coffee and alcoholic beverages.

Bowel Cleansing

Breuss writes in his book nothing about it; however, from my experience and based on study of various specialized literature on the subject, I would urge you to undergo bowel cleansing. With the end in mind that the bowels could perform their difficult work during fasting, they should be cleansed prior to treatment. There are various alternatives to doing this:

Chapter 6 - Important Tips on the Treatment

Glauber's Salt or Epsom Salt

You can get Glauber's or Epsom salt in a pharmacy. The first cleansing should be performed four days prior to the treatment and repeated in three days.

Proceed as follows: put one to three heaped teaspoons of the salt in a glass of lukewarm water (approx. 200-300 ml). Stir thoroughly and make sure that the crystals are fully dissolved. Shake up the mix with a spoon and drink it in one draught.

Important: do not take both salts during the treatment since they are not suitable as a regular laxative.

> **Tip:** *Glauber's or Epsom salt taste anything but nice. So prepare another glass of water in order to wash away the strong and salty taste.*

Mustard Seeds

Two or three days before the treatment take one tablespoon of mustard seeds a day after getting up. Subsequently drink a glass of lukewarm water and wait for the effect.

Sauerkraut Juice

Get at a Reformhaus shop a bottle of the sauerkraut juice that may be of value to you later. One or several glasses of it cleanse the bowels well.

For those who usually have no problems with a daily bowel evacuation, it will be sufficient to drink on the first day of the treatment one or two glasses of the sauerkraut juice just after getting up.

Chapter 6 - Important Tips on the Treatment

Enema

For a sensitive intestinal mucosa, an enema with lukewarm water or chamomile tea is better than the aforementioned practices. You will need a special device for this, the irrigator (pharmacy) and one or two liters of water or herbal tea, with a temperature of approx. 30-35 °C. Thus, the temperature of the liquid should be slightly less than the temperature of a human body to stimulate peristalsis – the muscle activity of the bowels.

Colon Hydrotherapy

This is in my opinion the most effective – but also the most complex - opportunity not only to cleanse the bowels but also to restore their normal functioning in good time before and during the Breuss Treatment.

> *Tip: if you read this book just out of interest, with no intention of undergoing this treatment you should nevertheless afford yourself the "luxury" and try just for once the colon hydrotherapy, thereby doing something good for your intestines.*

Information about this therapy as well as many other useful suggestions can be found on the Internet. For example on the website of the naturopathy practice Olaf Schultz-Friese, the address is in the appendix.

Preparation at Home

Sleep Place Investigation

After Breuss' experience most cancer patients sleep on top of so-called "earth rays" which are even more dangerous where they cross. Therefore, it makes sense to consult a "dowser" or

Chapter 6 - Important Tips on the Treatment

a "commuter" (addresses in the appendix) to look for these dangerous places in your apartment.
During this sleep place investigation it is particularly important that your bed stands on a "pure" place.

One may smile about it, but we have invited such experts to examine our bedroom and behold: under my bed, just under the prostate gland, was such a fault line. Of course, we did say the examination was necessary or for whom. So on the advice of experts we moved our beds half a meter aside - it is often sufficient to avoid a negative impact.

Now my wife and I sleep on a "pure" place.

Poison in Your Apartment

Rudolf Breuss warns very strongly about the presence in the apartment of hidden poisons such as:

- Naphthalene-based agents (mothballs etc.),
- Man-made camphor,
- DDT,
- Fly spray,
- Air purifiers in the toilet, etc.

These poisons are easy to recognize because of their strong, intensive smell. Remove these things from your home prior to the treatment and air the apartment thoroughly!

Organizational Preparation

1. Get a juice extractor or a kitchen appliance by which you are able to press juice. It must not be a high performance machine, but it should have sufficient power in order to

Chapter 6 - Important Tips on the Treatment

process the required vegetable varieties with ease. Perhaps, you will be able to borrow the appliance for six weeks from your friends or acquaintances?

2. In case of severe cancer (and what is "mild cancer"?) it is necessary, according to a recommendation made by Rudolf Breuss, to use <u>home-made</u> and <u>home-mixed</u> juices from organically-grown vegetables. Find a shop or market with organic goods and buy vegetables for the first few days (see Shopping list in Chapter 11).

3. If, for any reason, you cannot or do not want to prepare the juice <u>at home</u>, buy the corresponding quantity of ready-made juice. It is a maximum of 21 liters i.e. no more than 42 bottles (0.5 liter each) of the ready-made juice. But always remember: freshly pressed is always better than storable for two years. Note the section called "Making Your Own Vegetable Juice" in Chapter 8. In case you prefer ready-made juices, there will be no need, of course, to get a juice extractor.

4. Procure for the teas a letter scales or a kitchen scales <u>accurate to the gramme.</u>

5. Go to a pharmacy with the shopping list (Chapter 11) and order various teas for your type of cancer. You will find most teas there, and some in the Reformhaus shop. Some of them are even available only on prescription. In any event, I have had no getting them. Otherwise: Chapter 11, section "Procurement problems?"

6. <u>Do not let</u> the pharmacy or its suppliers mix the teas, but mix them on your own (see Chapter 10). In this case you

Chapter 6 - Important Tips on the Treatment

will know what the mix actually contains (for this reason you need the letter scales or accurate kitchen scales).

7. After three days at the most, various teas in your pharmacy should be available for collection; they will cost – as an indication – 100 to 120 Euros.

8. Mix the teas in accordance with your cancer type to store them for the next few days and weeks pursuant to Chapter 10.

I am referring to the following teas:

- **Kidney tea,** necessary in all types of cancer, the mix should be prepared only for the first three weeks,

- **Sage tea,** in Breuss' special tea mixture, necessary in all types of cancer. You can mix more of this tea in store as this tea mixture is one of the two most important drinks during the treatment,

- **Special tea mix** necessary in all types of cancer; thus, you can also prepare more of this mix as it is the second most important drink during the treatment.

When mixing the teas you can proceed, for example, in line with my recommendations for preparing the special tea mix in Chapter 10. As regards storage containers, Tupperware and similar tightly closing containers have proven their effectiveness.

Chapter 6 - Important Tips on the Treatment

9. Clearly label the teas mixed by you and also other teas and infusions foreseen for your treatment! You will find labels for most teas in the Appendix "Recommendations on Teas (Infusions) Preparation"; you can cut out or copy these labels and glue them to the corresponding containers so as to avoid confusion!

10. Prepare three or four drink containers, if you plan any activities outside your home during the treatment, for example, if you want or are obliged to work quite normally. These drink containers are required for various teas and juices while traveling. You can read more about this in this Chapter in the section called "On the Move during Cancer Treatment".

11. Craft for your motivation a "Control and reward model" (you will find my proposal for this in the Appendix "I did it!").

12. Copy the daily schedule (see Appendix) when possible, slightly enlarged, and attach it close to the place where you eat your meal, as a permanent memory aid, even though there will be nothing to eat there for 42 days.

13. On the eve of the treatment prepare two cups of kidney tea (Chapter 10). But do not drink the tea yet –you will start your treatment with this tea the next morning!

Are You Too Weak for the Treatment?

If, for the reasons explained in the previous chapter, you feel too weak to begin the treatment, the following applies:

Chapter 6 - Important Tips on the Treatment

1. Since the psyche of a patient plays an **important**, even decisive role for the success of the treatment, you should really want to undergo this course of treatment.

    Your goal should be to assimilate, think and clearly say:

    ### I want to beat the cancer!

2. You should not start the treatment immediately following an operation. Also, you need to wait for at least a month after chemotherapy. Breuss even recommends waiting at least two to five months, depending "on how the patient feels". I would say that in this case a balanced approach is important. I would reduce this waiting period, in exceptional cases, to a maximum of one month, before you get even weaker. What point is there in waiting if you are getting more feeble and infirm and have no alternative?

3. During this waiting period you should drink 1/16 liter (half a cup) of vegetable juice a day and eat lightly, for example, gruel soup, vegetable soup, vegetables and maybe chicken or veal or other light foods.

4. Drink vegetable juice in small sips (always well mixed with saliva!) before meals, together with the prescribed herbal teas, sage tea and kidney tea (see Chapter 10) like during cancer treatment.

5. Do not start the treatment until you feel strong enough.

6. Breuss recommends taking the Strath convalescent products immediately after treatment, so that the patient feels better much faster. Read a more detailed description

Chapter 6 - Important Tips on the Treatment

of these products below, in the sections "Fast Breaking" and "Readaptation". The same products should also be helpful during the preparation of a weakened patient for the Breuss Total Cancer Treatment. Thus, take a teaspoon of the Strath convalescent product three times a day, or two Bio-Strath yeast tablets.

7. During the treatment, also for weakened patients, it is **extremely important** that the patient moves himself or herself in fresh air. You will need a suitably gentle and slow rehabilitation program.

   And if movement in fresh air is no longer possible for you, you should at any rate take every opportunity to breathe in deeply fresh air outside for at least an hour a day.

During the Treatment

Blood Pressure, Sometimes Too High and Sometimes Too Low

During the treatment, you should always keep an eye on your blood pressure.

Blood pressure too high: in order to treat high blood pressure, you can follow the advice in the original Breuss book. It is also possible to drink in sips one or two cups of a cold yarrow tea per day and do the breathing exercises outlined by Breuss. Consuming brewer's or baker's yeast, in principle recommended by Breuss is, of course, not allowed during the treatment.

As a rule, however, blood pressure falls during the treatment anyhow.

Chapter 6 - Important Tips on the Treatment

I have high blood pressure, and prior to the treatment hypertension I had to take medicines. So, my blood pressure reached ideal values for me of 125: 75 during the treatment.

Blood pressure too low: for low blood pressure (generally defined as 110:60) Breuss recommends asking your doctor to prescribe you "something for the heart". Furthermore, he gives many general tips in his book (not only for the fight against cancer) which you can or should follow, apart from the things which are simply prohibited during the treatment, as, for example, eating celeriac salad or strawberries, which would otherwise be helpful.

I got one more **tip** on countering low blood pressure from alternative practitioners:
Drink two or three cups of Scotch broom tea per day. Scotch broom, synonym the common broom (Cytisus scoparius), earlier known as Sarothamnus scoparius, in medicine known as (Herba Spartii scoparii).

Preparation: some 2 grams of the herb are poured with hot water and left to infuse for 10 minutes.

Important: drink up to three cups a day at most of this infusion, no more.

Constipation

Possible constipation can be counteracted by various means. I would like to describe some of them below.

Background and consequences of constipation: if the digestive tract content is not transported away from your body as quickly as possible, waste products and toxins are retained in the body and absorbed into the blood as they had contact with

Chapter 6 - Important Tips on the Treatment

intestinal mucosa for too long.
It is often visible on the skin. It loses its natural colour, swells up, becomes oily, shiny and pimpled, or dry and matt; in short, the skin reacts to impurities.

Remedy: typically, it is possible to keep your intestines fit with a high-fiber, healthy diet and by drinking a lot of water. However, during the Breuss Treatment the body does not get these important high-fiber substances.

It is necessary, of course, to drink a lot in any case if you want to age in a healthy way, whether during the cancer treatment, or in normal everyday circumstances.

The intestine requires some assistance during the treatment in order to "flush out" accumulated waste products, superfluous parts of food and toxic substances.

Therefore, you should thoroughly and carefully empty the intestine as a preparation <u>before</u> the treatment. You can find a description of the corresponding methods in the section "Bowel Cleansing".

The general rule is that <u>during the treatment</u> emptying of the intestines should occur at the latest every third day.

Every patient decides on his/her own which of the following methods will be used to do this, if "nothing happens", as every person reacts differently to various opportunities.

In case of constipation, Rudolf Breuss advises:
- Make enemas using lukewarm (body temperature) water or chamomile tea,
- Or drink a mild laxative tea,

Chapter 6 - Important Tips on the Treatment

- Or gently insert a piece of hard butter into the anus.

My time-tested advice:
- A glass of bio-sauerkraut juice can often help.

Background: during the juice treatment, says Breuss, the blood in the portal vein circuit[5] becomes so stimulated that whatever is in the intestines is fully recycled by the body.

Therefore, it can happen that over a period of a few days the patient has hardly any bowel movements or even none at all, but suffers no discomfort.

Nevertheless, it is **important** that stool and urine are eliminated well, so that the decomposing substances do not stay for a long time in the body and not cause toxic effects.

Bad Breath and Body Odour

During treatment, the body egests toxins and waste products in large quantities. It occurs through all orifices of the body, i.e. also through the skin and mucous membranes in the mouth. Thus, this results in unpleasant body perspiration and bad breath.

What can we do about this?

Bad Breath

Is this the case, you can brush your teeth several times a day, also "between times". It is also possible to gently brush your tongue with a tongue scraper.

---

5) The portal vein circuit is a vein (Vena portae). Its task is to bring nutrients contained in the intestines, and also possible toxins, directly to the liver. The latter are then degraded in the liver before they reach further bloodstream.

Chapter 6 - Important Tips on the Treatment

Gargling with a mouth wash can also help you to get rid of bad breath for some time.

And what about using chewing gum for this purpose? It is a very bad idea! Breuss does not address this point, though, but the facts speak against chewing.

1. The masticator movements send signals to the stomach, which sound something like this: "Attention, now there will be food!". The stomach sets itself up for an intake of food – unfortunately, in vain! Consequence: the stomach begins to rumble, the sensation of hunger appears, and we really do not want this to happen during the Breuss Treatment.

2. Chewing gums contain, along with sweeting agents, many synthetic substances that we do not need during treatment. After all, our aim is to <u>load off, purify and detoxify</u> the body. Thus, it doesn't make a lot of sense to burden it with additional substances.

Body Odour

By taking a bath or shower more often you can prevent fellow human beings turning their noses up when they contact you directly.
So why not do something at the same time for your joints, as I thoroughly describe in the book "Rudolf Breuss Fasting Method...Simply Ingenious" (see Bibliography)? The "self-prescribed" bath treatment has been very good for my joints and me!
Those who during daily sport activities in the fresh air actively inhale and exhale, can properly feel how their "stale air" escapes into the surrounding air and they feel fresher with

Chapter 6 - Important Tips on the Treatment

every step. At the same time, by running or walking, they spur their skin on to excrete toxins through sweat so that their oral mucosa gets less to do with eliminating toxins.

Headache

Sometimes during treatment, especially in the first three or four days, headaches occur. They might be caused by various reasons:

Insufficient Bowel Movements

Most waste products and toxins are eliminated from the body during treatment through the intestines. It is, therefore, important that the bowels before the treatment (see section "Bowel Cleansing", Chapter 6) are cleansed and thereby emptied. During treatment the bowels should be thoroughly emptied at least every three days (see sections "Constipation/ Bowel Movements" in Chapter 6).

Considering that during treatment the intestines receive no dietary fibre, which normally ensures good digestion, one of the possibilities for bowel movements mentioned in these sections should help the intestines. This is very important because if you fail to do this it can result in retoxication of the body.

Potential consequences: headache, weakness and even depression.

Not Drinking Enough

Although the quantities of teas to be taken during treatment are more or less determined, the quantity of sage tea and the special tea mix is very flexible. You should drink both teas as

Chapter 6 - Important Tips on the Treatment

much as possible. The point is that at the beginning of the Breuss Treatment the body is very dehydrated, and simultaneously self-cleaning actions of the body occur as to rinsing out of waste products and toxins, and both drinks enter the body's circulatory system.

This temporarily increased concentration of breakdown products in the body can be a trigger for headaches. The more toxins that need to be broken down the longer that the headaches will endure. Unfortunately, the stronger the headaches will be.

High fluid intake comes to the rescue. It ensures that waste products and toxins are eliminated from the body as quickly as possible.

Hence, at the beginning of treatment, it is advisable to use high a dosage of the sage tea in the special Breuss tea mixture and of the tea special mix rather than low dosage!

Too Much Stress

Stress is generally harmful to the body during fasting and can cause headaches. The Breuss Treatment not only fights cancer but also assists in regenerating the whole body. The immune system should be strengthened, and headaches caused by stress are counterproductive.

It would be best, of course, if you could take time out for treatment, be it from one's job, or from housekeeping. Where this is not possible, one should try - for example – autogenic training, for relaxation. Increased activities in the fresh air, such as sports or extensive walks could help to overcome stress.

Chapter 6 - Important Tips on the Treatment

Withdrawal Symptoms

As is generally known, all stimulants during fasting are taboo – including beloved coffee. Those who are used to regularly drinking a lot of coffee in everyday life can in the first days suffer from severe headaches because of the lack of coffee. Fortunately, the body becomes disaccustomed to coffee after several days, and the headaches subside.

As a preventive measure, it would be much better to reduce the coffee drinking one or two weeks before the treatment, slowly and controlled, to zero, than to stop it abruptly in the first day of fasting.
Smokers will have, of course, the same problem as coffee drinkers but on a different level.

Out in the Fresh Air!

During treatment it is very **important** to move oneself into fresh air. Rudolf Breuss talks about it briefly and succinctly: "It is good to have a lot of exercise in the fresh air!"

In the autumn of 2003 I took to Nordic Walking and throughout the whole treatment I walked around 3.5 km in the fresh air a day. During the entire treatment I walked the respectable distance of 120 km!

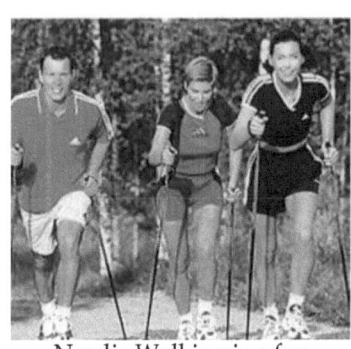

Nordic Walking is a fun

I can highly recommend Nordic Walking as a sporting activity for the period of treatment! It is easy to learn; moreover, it is an effective training exercise for the whole body, with additional load on the stomach, chest and arm muscles.

You choose your speed depending on how you feel. Thanks to this, you can also actively move in the fresh air with impaired performance.

Even at a relatively low speed, through the arm action, the heart frequency and transformation of energy are increased, so that the burning of calories compared to normal walking increases by 40%.

One more advantage is relief of the back and knee and foot joints. Besides, through Nordic Walking and use of special poles, muscle tensions in the shoulder and neck areas are loosened.

If you want to learn Nordic Walking, ask in your sports club or a sporting goods shop about possible introductory courses, since one should exercise this sport in the right way from the beginning.

Vegetable Juice and Additional Juices

If you cannot stand vegetable juices, then my advice and tips as to the juices potentially help so that you will even be able to undergo this treatment. For further information, please refer to Chapter 8, the section "If you don't like vegetable juice (anymore)".

In addition to the vegetable juice, writes Breuss, the patient may have a mouthful of sauerkraut juice every now and again.

To avoid monotony of the treatment during its last critical

Chapter 6 - Important Tips on the Treatment

days, drinking of a little lemon juice is also allowed, but <u>never apple juice</u>. Exception: freshly squeezed apple juice is allowed in between *by itself*, <u>but never</u> mixed with other juices. And no sugar! These juices should be drunk in sips, mixing them well with saliva.

But be careful! Use these tips sparingly. In fact, I am talking about the means which will help you to overcome the "deadlock" in the last week. See Appendix "The 35th Day".

Smoking

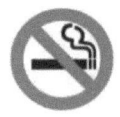

"Cancer patients who do not give up smoking for good", writes Breuss briefly and concisely, "will not benefit from my juice treatment at all!"

Eating and Drinking Beyond Medical Prescriptions

The question that comes up repeatedly from patients is whether they can eat, apart from the juice diet, *a little bread, honey, eggs or vegetables*. Or whether they can drink *e.g. black currant, raspberry or pumpkin juice.*

Rudolf Breuss answers such questions unambiguously:

NO!

Drinking Water

It is probably self-evident today that it is necessary to use where possible only "good" water for the preparation of teas (read more about this in Chapter 7 "Strengthening the Immune System").

Chapter 6 - Important Tips on the Treatment

Earlier the water quality was not yet an issue, otherwise Rudolf Breuss would have dedicated several sentences to this sensitive topic. Thus, in his book – the original edition of 1990 – he does not address the issue of water at all. He mentions neither water as such nor the question as to whether patients can drink water apart from the teas. So, he does not allow them to drink clear water during treatment.

But he keeps saying that patients should drink the sage tea in the Breuss tea mixture and in the special tea mix as much as they want and the more, the better.

In my opinion, water would only water down the effect of herbal teas by diluting the vital teas, and the patient would receive fewer ingredients.

In other words: each glass of glass would mean one cup sage tea or special tea mix less. And this would be counterproductive for the success of the treatment.

Injections, Chemotherapy, Radiotherapy and Drugs

During treatment patients **must not receive** injections, chemotherapy or radiation; they should also **refrain**, according to Breuss, from previously administered drugs. However, on the issue of drugs, he makes an exception: diabetics should continue their insulin treatment.

Here I would like to add my experiences from several joint fastings: I have seen how patients with type II diabetes underwent the Breuss Treatment without taking their medication. After three weeks of treatment the intermediate examinations showed such values that the doctors asked with astonishment what had the patients actually done. These values were better than ever in the last 20 years.

Chapter 6 - Important Tips on the Treatment

Normal Work during Cancer Treatment

During treatment, according to Breuss, bed rest is not necessary in most cases. On the contrary, one should work if possible, in order to switch off from the thoughts about food and illness.

I can only confirm this – not only was work during treatment good for me, but it also gave me a lot of fun.

Below is a short list of things I did during treatment:

- Initially it was work as executive director of a small computer support firm (whose office was in the house where I live – which of course made a lot of things easier) with all the duties associated with these activities.

- In addition, there was a construction of an herb spiral in the garden with its really strenuous dimensions (total weight of some 7.5 tons, and that is as much as 7, 500 kg!). The spiral had a diameter of about 3 m, and above ground level of 110 cm.

  There is information how to build such a spiral in the Internet, e.g. on the website www.kraeuterei.de (and then click "Kräuterspirale").

Of course, there is a whole range of books about it. Thus, during treatment one is not "weak in the legs". As for me, I certainly was not.

Chapter 6 - Important Tips on the Treatment

- All in all, I can say from my own experience: during treatment I was able to perform my duties in and out of home without any reductions – in most cases even more and better than I normally do, simply because I was feeling fine.

- In my leisure time I was also able to carry out my voluntary functions and obligations as chairman of a traditional club – as always and with pleasure.

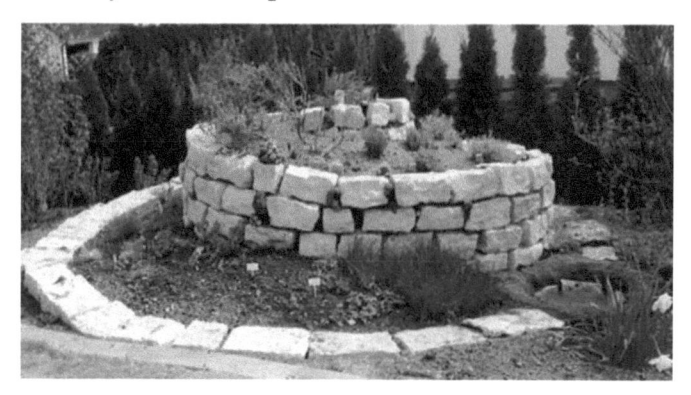

Built by myself

From other participants of the Breuss Total Cancer Treatment I know that they have released innumerable endorphins during the entire treatment, also called "happiness hormones". They not only felt well but they also worked more than usual.

An acquaintance of mine, an independent businessman, for example, took great care of his family (something he had never done before) starting from breakfast which he prepared for everybody, to lunch which he cooked and lovingly served and to a festive dinner party so that his family had the impression they were staying in a five star Hilton hotel. And all this without having taken even a morsel for himself!! In addition,

Chapter 6 - Important Tips on the Treatment

he worked in his supermarket not experiencing this work as a burden. His employees admitted frankly that their boss has never before been so mild-tempered and friendly as during his cancer treatment.
This is what the happiness hormones can cause...

With respect to another businessman, also an acquaintance of mine, a master craftsman, I know that during treatment he extended his normal working day - consciously or unconsciously - of 12 hours to 15 hours on average. He was constantly on the move, meeting his potential and actual customers, and nevertheless he did not feel stressed.

He simply enjoyed his work during the cancer treatment. He was calm, level-headed and concentrated and worked effectively and efficiently. No traces of distraction or minimizing labour due to the treatment.

Cancer Treatment on the Move

Preparation of juice and tea takes place mainly early in the morning, or, alternatively, in the evening.

All morning, and after your excellent "lunch" – a plate of onion broth ☻ - for the entire afternoon you can move wherever you wish, as well as work provided that you take along several thermoses (bottles) of home-made drinks.

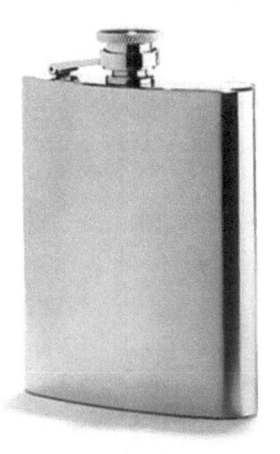

Chapter 6 - Important Tips on the Treatment

Here are the recommendations that I personally tested:

- A small thermos (bottle, hip flask, etc.) with a maximum capacity of ¼ liter (and a daily stock of 0.5 liter) for vegetable juice,

- Another thermos for cranesbill (Herb Robert) tea,

- One thermos for the special tea mix which is to be alternated with sage tea. This flask can be large enough since these tea mixtures can be consumed in any desirable quantity.

- One thermos for onion broth,

- The fifth container with a capacity of ¼ liter can be used for additional cancer-specific tea that you may need to drink throughout the day,

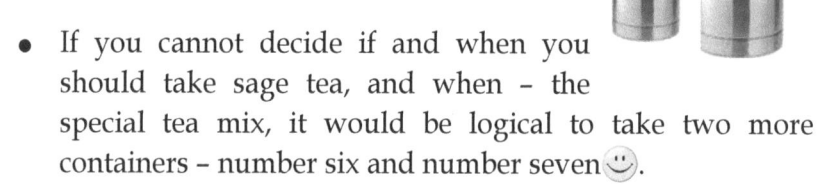

- If you cannot decide if and when you should take sage tea, and when – the special tea mix, it would be logical to take two more containers – number six and number seven ☺.

(Short) Trips during Cancer Treatment

Sometimes, during a 42-day course of cancer treatment, you have to make short trips lasting several days (but not weeks, otherwise you have chosen the wrong time frame for treatment!). If this is the case, keep following my recommendations above, introducing slight modifications if required:

Chapter 6 - Important Tips on the Treatment

- Containers and thermos flasks used for various teas must be larger, as you will have to take enough tea to keep you going for several days. Since tea is normally consumed cold, there is no need to prepare it during the trip.

- However, if your trip lasts for more than three or four days, you will have to take dry herbs and mixtures to be able to prepare fresh tea.

- In the hotel kitchen there will certainly be a possibility to have onion broth cooked. That can also apply to herbal teas (will tips provide additional motivation?).

- As it will hardly be possible to press fresh vegetable juice every day (after all, who would want to carry a juice extractor on a business trip?), you will have to drink ready-made vegetable juice.

Happiness Hormones...

During cancer treatment – just like any fasting therapy – after three to five days patients experience a release of endorphins, so-called "happiness hormones", and serotonin. Due to that, patients undergoing fasting therapy feel completely at ease and do not feel hungry. Many patients also report a reduction in pain during fasting, which also has a positive effect on their mood[6].

---

6) Happiness hormones is the term for several neurotransmitters (substances that relay information from one nerve cell to another):
Endorphins control the sensations of pain and hunger. They directly influence the production of sex hormones; secretion of endorphins leads to feelings of euphoria. Endorphinergic system is activated, among others, in emergency situations.
Serotonin is produced in the central nervous system, liver, spleen and intestinal mucosa from the amino acid L-tryptophan. Balanced or slightly elevated serotonin levels evoke feelings of comfort or contentment.

Chapter 6 - Important Tips on the Treatment

By the way, an effect similar to that of fasting is attributed only to psychotropic or narcotic substances like ecstasy. The thing is, fasting reduces stress, opens new perspectives and introduces major changes to the patient's perception of the world. In many cases, therapeutic fasting produces a relaxing and calming effect on people's behavior in their everyday lives. Cancer treatment may therefore trigger profound lifestyle changes.

Positive experience acquired through cancer treatment often brings about a health-conscious lifestyle, as fasting in our hectic time is a kind of reflection and revisiting, a certain introversion.

Cancer treatment can also turn out to be a stimulus for developing a conscious approach to healthy nutrition and weight loss.

After Treatment: Taking Control of Success

Diagnostic Procedures

If you wish to make sure that you have beaten cancer, you can wait for about two weeks after the end of the course of treatment and then undergo a medical check-up. That's the time interval advised by Rudolf Breuss, as the body obviously needs some time to readjust before it produces meaningful values.

The range and details of health check procedures should be discussed with your doctor. As a rule, the check-up is restricted

Source: Wikipedia

Chapter 6 - Important Tips on the Treatment

to the control of **blood values** focusing on **tumor markers**[7] (up to 20 various values). This applies to all types of cancer.

In case of bladder and prostate cancers, relatively accurate results can be obtained, in particular, in contrast to the **PSA test** (see page 112), using the **DiaPat method** (www.diapat.com) whereby any risks for the patient are very low.

Disputable Diagnostic Procedures

If your doctor wants to use other diagnostic methods in order to find out whether you are healed, you must know the following details:

The need for a **CT scan** has, in my opinion, to be carefully weighed up, since one CT scan involves radiation exposure which is 1,000 (!) times higher than, for example, an x-ray examination. The radiation a patient receives during one chest CT scan is equal to the radiation he or she would receive from a series of one x-ray examination conducted in the morning, at noon and in the evening - **for a whole year**!

---

7) <u>Tumor markers</u> are proteins which build up in the body during development and growth of malignant tumors, i.e. of cancer. They can be measured in blood or other body fluids. An elevated concentration of these tumor markers may indicate an oncology disease or recurrent cancer, a so-called recurrence. Tumor markers are very important for keeping the results of tumor treatment under control after surgery or chemotherapy. Besides, a further rise of tumor markers in blood may indicate a possible recurrence. Based on tumor markers, a doctor can detect such recurrence at an early stage and immediately start the necessary therapy. On the other hand, if the check-up shows a drop in tumor marker level below a certain value, this means that cancer has been beaten.

Source: State Medical Council of Baden-Württemberg

Chapter 6 - Important Tips on the Treatment

Patients fail to recognize the danger, as many physicians play down radiation hazards, or know far too little about it[8]. Often enough, physicians responsible for treatment financially participate in the CT device and have to ensure its profitability.

A need for **biopsy**, with its inaccurate results, conducted in order to determine the success of the treatment, is also rather disputable. I would not perform these examinations.

What can surely be recommended for diagnostics, is **magnetic resonance therapy** (MRT). The only question that arises in this respect is whether this high-tech expenditure is necessary, particularly in view of the fact that many physicians use this ultra-modern device to make extra money (see above) and so try to operate it as often as possible. Without any particular benefit for you.

In case of prostate cancer, urologists mainly prefer the controversial **PSA-test**. As the science journalist Dr. Klaus Koch, who specializes in PSA, points out, *"The test is unreliable because of its high false-positive rate."* ((Ed.: it means the patient is healthy but the test falsely identifies him or her as sick). *According to the "Deutsches Ärzteblatt" (German Medical Journal) for 2006, the false-positive rate is 75%.* (Ed.: it means that 75% of patients are healthy, while their test results are positive!). This makes the test not only pointless, but plain dangerous: psychological consequences have an enormous impact on falsely diagnosed men." In the meantime, for me the PSA screening is "dead". **Those who will still choose to do it, must know that despite its positive result, three out of four patients are healthy!**

---

8)   I received this information from the spokesman of the Ruhr University in Bochum, Dr. Josef König, and also from the ZDF-show "Frontal 21" of 15th May 2007. Read more on Wikipedia.

Chapter 6 - Important Tips on the Treatment

Question at the End of Treatment: Am I Healed Now?

As you will find out in this section, it is not that easy to give a valid answer to the question above. If you were to ask me whether I am healthy, I will reply with utter conviction and a resounding YES. And that has been the case for the past nine years.

Viewed realistically, the outcome of the Breuss treatment can only be determined as successful in five years' time. This timeframe – five years – is seen by oncologists as an important yardstick, because after this period there is a strong probability that if a former cancer patient has no complaints, he/she has been cured. At least, that's the point of view of oncology.

Many cancer patients who were treated entirely by methods of conventional medicine, live in constant fear of metastases and relapses. Surprisingly enough, I must state that people who managed to beat cancer with the Breuss treatment, are mostly free of fear. Perhaps it's because the 42-day fasting is virtually a healing in itself, and it carries with it a profound change in consciousness – in any case, it is a good feeling!

A check-up designed to make sure that you have beaten cancer with The Cure, is generally the responsibility of conventional medicine. Therefore, let us first examine whether we, or somebody treated by means of conventional medicine, will ever hear that he or she was healed.

It is not very likely that you will hear the sentence "You

are cured from cancer" from a doctor working within the framework of conventional medicine. Here is an excerpt dealing with this issue from "Frankfurter Allgemeine" of 20.4.2012. I quote verbatim:

Temporary Cure?

According to the most recent projections of the Robert Koch Institute in Berlin, this year 486,000 people in Germany will develop cancer. It means 1,331 newly diagnosed cases every day. Many of them will survive the disease by years and decades thanks to effective medical treatment. The Robert Koch Institute currently estimates the number of people diagnosed with cancer more than 10 years ago, at 2,1 million persons. Medicine speaks quite soberly of long-time survivors. *(My comment: based on my observations, the word "cured" does not exist in medical oncology. The best result ever is "long-time survivors"! This category includes persons who have survived a surgery conducted by means of conventional medicine by five years from the date of original diagnosis).* But are these people really cured, or do they suffer more than it used to be believed, from long-term effects and psychological trauma caused by their cancer experience? This year's congress of the German Society for Internal Medicine in Wiesbaden attempted to find an answer to this question. Georgia Schilling from the Hubertus Wald Tumor Center at the Hamburg-Eppendorf University Medical Center put forward the opinion that medium-term and long-term effects should be given more attention. *"53% of long-time survivors report health problems"*, said the oncologist in Wiesbaden. *"49% complain about non-medical problems. For many survivors, five years after they got rid of tumor, the disease is not over yet".* Dr. Schilling mentioned a number of potential delayed effects. Some cytotoxins from chemotherapy cause

Chapter 6 - Important Tips on the Treatment

damage to heart, lungs, kidneys, hormone system and the gastrointestinal tract, so that associated diseases of these organs must be taken into account. New biological therapies can often take years, which makes cancer therapy a rather long process. Little is known about their delayed effects since many biologics *(Ed.: biologics should target the processes inside human body)* have been used for only a few years. Likewise, radiation treatment or surgery can have side effects. Depending on the type of tumor, women are more likely to develop an early menopause. Many patients develop osteoporosis, chronic fatigue, bone or phantom pains, numbness, sensitivity disorders, discomfort; some patients can have no more children. They can also develop secondary tumors arising from initial treatment, or caused by advanced age. Also, according to Georgia Schilling, one should not underestimate the psychological consequences of cancer experience. Many patients live in constant fear of a relapse and are no longer able to work. Some of them have to cope with impaired memory, concentration, learning ability and coordination. *(My comment: do you understand now why conventional medicine chooses not to use the word "cured"?)*

Numerous Consequences

Women who have been treated for cancer at the age of 15-35, have fewer children than those who have had no oncological diseases. Due to the treatment they have undergone, these women either lose their fertility or do not feel strong and healthy enough to raise children. Thus, a cancerous disease can call into question the patient's life design. Dr. Schilling also reported that cancer patients have to receive medical treatment for depression twice as often as their peers who do not have cancer. The former are also less inclined to live a healthy lifestyle. *"In a survey, 36% of long-time survivors described their health as poor"*, reported an

Chapter 6 - Important Tips on the Treatment

oncologist in Wiesbaden, *"58% are overweight, 23% smoke, 82% do not eat the recommended amounts of vegetables and fruit, and only one out of two people pursues physical activity on a regular basis"*.

As to cancer in children and adolescents whereby the survival rates with an average of 80% are very high, experts in this field have longer experience of dealing with the delayed organic effects of the therapy, primarily with the risk of secondary tumors. Alexander Katalinic from the Institute of Cancer Epidemiology at the University of Lьbeck, speaking in Wiesbaden, referred to the epidemiological data provided by the National Cancer Institute in the US, according to which the risk of a secondary tumor in persons who had a tumor before the age of 18, is six times higher. Those who were treated for cancer at the age of 18-29, have a threefold higher risk of a therapy-related secondary tumor, said Katalinic. Medical science has virtually ignored many other problems of long¬-term survival in adolescents and young adults.

---End of quote

Conventional Medicine Avoids Using the Word "Cured"

Do you understand now why your doctor will hardly say to you, "The Breuss treatment cured you"? In fact, he chooses not to say these words even after surgery, radiation or chemotherapy conducted by means of conventional medicine before a period of five to ten years has passed. Instead of "healthy" or "cured", the doctor prefers to speak of remission (in medicine it means a temporary or permanent subsiding of clinical symptoms). Here, differentiation is made between:
- Complete remission (the notion closest to "cured")
- Partial remission (e.g., 50% reduction in tumor volume)
- Minimal remission (25-50% reduction in tumor volume).

What I Did – and What I Wish I Had Done

After treatment, I restricted myself merely to laboratory analyses and blood tests. In those days, I had great trust in PSA levels. Be that as it may. My priority is to feel healthy and cured. That is the key. As long as the tumor markers do not rise, I am objectively healthy – and I will never be talked into thinking otherwise. By anyone. If, contrary to expectations, the values which I check once a year displayed noticeable and continuous growth, I would simply repeat the course of treatment, maybe even twice.

Fast Breaking and Readaptation

Preliminary Remarks

After the last day of the Breuss treatment, it is necessary to slowly adjust your body to a 'normal' diet.

Chapter 6 - Important Tips on the Treatment

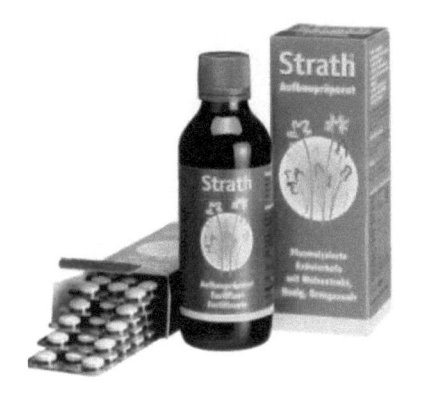

The body should switch to its regular nutrition program and energy metabolism, whereby it receives strength and energy from digestion. This process has to be slow and gradual.

Right after the therapy, for two to four weeks, Breuss recommends to continue drinking some 1/16 liter (about ½ cup) of vegetable juice per day in small sips before meals. For this, I would recommend ready-made juice as taking into account a small quantity of 1/16 liter, i.e. 62.5 ml – less than half a coffee cup – there is no point in pressing juice at home.

For faster recovery, Breuss advises a teaspoon of the Strath Elixir (convalescent product) to be taken three times a day, or two Strath yeast tablets to be likewise taken three times a day. This convalescent product consists of herbal yeast. It can be taken for several months or until the patient feels well again.

Practical tip: liquid herbal yeast can be mixed with vegetable juice. However, not during treatment but only before and after it, to revitalize your body.

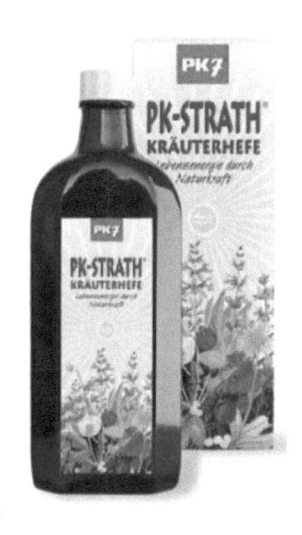

For details of where to purchase these products, see the appendix and the "Shopping List".

Chapter 6 - Important Tips on the Treatment

The golden rule when fasting is to provide the body with enough time to break the fast and readjust to a normal diet – about one third of the duration of the treatment – since during fasting it received no nourishment. When applied to the Breuss treatment, it means that after the treatment, 14 days should be dedicated to readaptation. Should the treatment – for any reason whatsoever - be discontinued prematurely, this rule will still apply.

The matter is that cancer treatment causes the body to stop producing gastric juices and inhibits intestinal activity.

Therefore, the return to normal digestion should not be too abrupt, otherwise it will cause stomach cramps or even severe damage to the digestive system.

Thus, you have to observe iron discipline and patiently readjust your body to solid food.

Breaking Your Fast

So, you complete the Breuss treatment on the 42nd day of fasting. On this day, go to the market and buy everything you need for breaking the fast and for the first readaptation day:

ripe, fragrant apples, bananas, potatoes, carrots, a small leek, some celery, raisins, finely sliced almonds and almond cream. If you do not have yeast flakes (sold at a health food store), fresh or dried herbs as oregano, parsley, marjoram, possibly also nutmeg at home or in the garden, you ought to buy them,

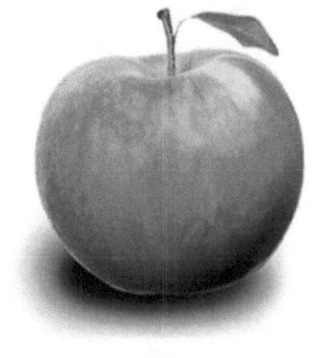

Chapter 6 - Important Tips on the Treatment

too. Slightly stale bread (or roll) rounds off your shopping list. You will see: these purchases will be highly enjoyable!

Your fast breaking starts the next day: at breakfast, reward yourself for your self-control with a solemn fast-breaking ceremony during which you will slowly, using all your senses – those of sight, touch, smell and taste – eat a ripe, fresh apple. Peel and quarter an apple, grate two quarters of it into thin threads. Enjoy this freshly grated apple by the spoonful and chew each mouthful slowly and thoroughly.

Do take your time over this…

In most cases, half an apple will be sufficient to start with, because after six weeks of fasting the need for food is still very low. Besides, take at least two or three big cups of tea of your choice (herbal or fruit), drinking it in small sips.

In the course of the morning feel free to eat, bite by bite, a slightly stale roll – as always, it must be chewed well.

As to lunch, a good solution will be vegetable broth with "dressing". Slightly steam chopped potatoes, carrots, celery and leek, pour some water and simmer gently for 15 minutes. Then add vegetable broth, half a teaspoon of yeast flakes and herbs, and your first "genuine" post fast soup is ready. Enjoy it slowly, with tranquility and contemplation.

Please make fresh home-made soup and stay away from any packet soups.

From time to time, drink water or tea. You may consider giving up dairy products over the next few weeks (according to the motto, "No animal products"). Read more on this in Chapter 7, section "Protein Revisited".

In the evening you can eat, for example, one steamed potato and some stewed carrot.

Post-treatment Day Two can be started with porridge: cook 3 tablespoons of oat flakes in two cups of water with a tiny pinch of salt until tender. Then add some grated apple, a few raisins, one tablespoon finely sliced almonds, one teaspoon of almond cream and maybe one more fruit variety. Mix well and eat while still warm – bon appétit!

In the evening, drink two to three cups of herbal tea. You should take your evening meal at 18.00 at the latest, otherwise your sleep can be disturbed by digestion.

Just like on the preceding days, carry out your daily physical activities, but avoid excessive physical exertion. Give yourself a little rest after meals.

Readaptation

On the following days, you should start slowly adjusting your body to the type of diet which you will stick to in future, be it vegetarian, flexitarian (flexitarians or semi-vegetarians eat a mostly vegetarian diet, but occasionally enjoy a good piece of meat, like a traditional family Sunday roast), be it a calorie-reduced or a stimulant free diet (a diet free from tea, coffee, alcohol and tobacco).

Additionally, here is the list of general rules and instructions to be followed on readaptation days:

Additionally, here is the list of general rules and instructions

Chapter 6 - Important Tips on the Treatment

to be followed on readaptation days:

- Listen to yourself, monitor changes in your body.
- You can experience a slight drop in performance, this is due to the restoration of your gut function.
- On readaptation days drink at least two to three liters of herbal or fruit tea (not necessarily your remaining Breuss teas, although they will do not harm), water, unsweetened juices, but no alcohol, coffee or black tea.
- Do not drink during meals, only before or after them, in order not to dilute your digestive juices which to this point are rather scarce.
- If possible, on readaptation days stick to your sports program in the fresh air. However, you should not exert yourself – let your body regain its strength.
- Additionally, on readaptation days do not let anything distract you from eating, be it reading, music, conversations or TV, and enjoy food with all your senses – sight, smell and taste.
- On readaptation days, prepare food and drink juices with no salt. Otherwise, water retention will cause the tissues to bloat. The fast has restored your taste buds and made them more sensitive to all the taste nuances of natural food, so you do not need any flavor enhancers.
- Try to eat food rich in fibre, gradually integrating into your diet raw vegetables, healthy cereals such as wheat bran or flaxseed; choose fish over meat, eat light and freshly prepared potato and vegetable soups, dairy products and easily digestible food.

Chapter 6 - Important Tips on the Treatment

- On readaptation days, eat small portions as your stomach has been reduced. However, you will be surprised at just how quickly the sensation of fullness will emerge.

- Chew slowly and carefully.

- Make sure your food and drinks are consumed at a stomach-friendly temperature – neither too hot, nor too cold.

- On readaptation days, you do not need additional stimulants to encourage bowel movements, instead, wait for natural bowel movements.

- The absence of bowel movements should not be perceived as a cause for worry. A glass of kefir, yogurt or lukewarm water taken before breakfast will help solve the problem. Another good home remedy in this case will also be blackthorn tea made from its blossom or leaves (health food store).

- Prepare this tea in the following way: boil two teaspoons of blackthorn blossom or blackthorn leaves in a quarter liter of water and pass them through a sieve. Two cups of this tea will produce the desired effect.

- You can stimulate natural intestinal peristalsis by adding a few flax seeds to your food.

- Avoid the use of laxatives during this period, they will not do you any good as they will make your intestines even more inert.

- On readaptation days, just like during the treatment, take time out for yourself after meals. Lie down for digestion.

- On readaptation days, avoid stress and mental strain.

- On readaptation days, just like during the treatment,

Chapter 6 - Important Tips on the Treatment

working out without excessive physical exertion will do you good.

- On the 14th day of readaptation you officially complete your cancer treatment. You feel rejuvenated, purified and healthy.

If you want to read more about the transition from fasting to solid food, I would recommend you read the book by Dr. med. Hellmut Lützner and Hellmut Million, "Eating Right After Fasting" (see Bibliography).

Our New Diet

In general, our diet, at least with regard to breakfast and pre-lunchtime, is quite in line with the still topical program Fit fürs Leben / Fit for Life based on the book by H. Diamond (see Bibliography).

Our menu consists primarily of freshly cooked food with as little salt as possible. We enjoy tasty and healthy food and realize the importance of thorough chewing aimed at stimulating its digestion in our body.

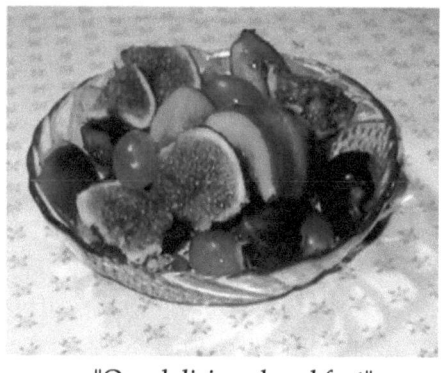

"Our delicious breakfast"

...and this is what our menu looks like:

For breakfast we usually eat fruit beautifully sliced into fruit salad. That means no rolls, no bread, no butter, no margarine, no honey and no marmalade or jam. Only

Chapter 6 - Important Tips on the Treatment

fruit. Served with delicious herbal tea from various regions around the world (my wife's choice) and a cup of coffee (my choice).

Between breakfast and lunch, we again eat nothing but fruit, for example, an apple or two, sometimes three or four.

Occasionally, the Thomars have brunch – in the form of half a roll, sometimes even a whole roll.

At the same time, we do not slavishly adhere to these self-imposed rules: in a hotel, on trips or on vacations, we can "afford" to eat an extensive buffet breakfast.

For lunch we eat (even) more vegetables, (even) less meat (no more than once a week, like flexitarians).

As to pork, we have completely eliminated it from our diet. We prefer meat directly from farmers, based on the motto "You've got to spoil yourself sometimes", but instead of meat, we often eat fish for lunch or dinner.

For dinner the Thomars eat cheese, from time to time sausage (made of beef or poultry, not pork). All of these are local foods and come straight from the farmer or local butcher, with fish, preferably salt-water fish, not thermally processed, i.e. boiled or fried, etc., for example, soused herring, Bismarck herring or rollmop.

We usually avoid coffee, black and green tea, preferring instead herbal and fruit tea.

However, we do not abstain from our daily Espresso after meals and can occasionally pamper ourselves with cappuccino or latte macchiato.

Chapter 6 - Important Tips on the Treatment

A Hearth of Your Own Is Worth Gold

Does this proverb also apply to microwave ovens and induction cookers

Microwave Ovens - Perfect Vitamin Killers

Please, do not think that we do not have a modern kitchen. Here you will find all kinds of appliances such as a refrigerator, glass ceramic cooker, even a steam/baking oven, and surely a dishwasher.

What you won't (any longer) find here, however, is our very own "nuclear power plant" (which applies to our microwave oven). Several years ago we banished it to the basement and later disposed of it. Why? See the answer below[9].

What is definitely known is that a microwave oven destroys plant secondary compounds in vegetables that are so valuable for maintaining good health.

This fact has been recently established by Spanish researchers. They tested it with the aid of broccoli, which is considered a

---

9) What radar engineers consider the most dangerous of all forms of energy, is seen in household equipment as perfectly harmless:
Microwaves (high-frequency radiation). Cellular phones have more so-called leakage radiation, says a household technologist. According to him, microwave ovens become dangerous only when the front panel gets broken – in this case, the stove may start irradiating the hand instead of a chicken. In contrast to the electric stove, you may not notice it immediately, but only when you start to feel painful burns under the skin.
The Swiss biologist Hans Hertel also considers microwaves hazardous to health: in his opinion, microwave ovens cause cancer. For his statements, he was even summoned to court in the 1990s, and acquitted by the European Court of Human Rights.
Some scientists believe microwaves to be dangerous since the irradiation they use causes food molecules to vibrate. How this affects the human body is still unknown.

Source: Bavarian Radio, Channel B5 Health,
http://www.br-online.de/umwelt-gesundheit/artikel/0511/13-mikrowelle/index.xml

Chapter 6 - Important Tips on the Treatment

particularly healthy vegetable. Its ingredients are believed to have a preventive effect against cancer – but only if not cooked in a microwave.

Research conducted by the University of Murcia has proved that when microwaved, vegetables lose much of their healthy substances. Most importantly, microwaving destroys antioxidants, which protect our body from cancer.

Microwaves destroy almost 100% of flavonoids, 87% of caffeic acid derivatives and 74% of sinapic acid.

Gentle steaming on a conventional oven largely preserves all these nutrients.

Particularly sensitive to microwave radiation is vitamin B12, with typical losses of 30%-40%.

Chapter 6 - Important Tips on the Treatment

Do Induction Stoves Place a Pregnant Woman and Fetus at Risk?

The next issue is the induction cooker. These appliances heat a cooking vessel through magnetic induction by using alternating magnetic fields which induce alternating electric currents in electrical conductors.

The design of these stoves makes it inevitable that some part of these magnetic fields is also released to the environment, including to those persons who are nearby.

In view of the fact that the human body also belongs in the sense described above to "electrical conductors", these magnetic fields also induce currents inside the human body.

The intensity of electric currents increases with the strength of the magnetic field (which is similar to conventional electric cookers) and its frequency, which is up to a thousand times higher than in conventional electric cookers.
Thus, induced currents will be higher by the same factor.

The best known health effect of low frequency magnetic fields is causing (or triggering) childhood leukemia. According to the Technical Institute for Electromagnetic Compatibility with Environment[10], the danger also exists that induction cookers cause the same effect.
The experts of this Institute advise, in particular, pregnant women against using induction cookers.

---

10)   Source: Report on Electrosmog, April 2002. The question about potential risks caused by exposure to induction cookers was answered by Dr. Peter Nießen from the Technical Institute for Electromagnetic Compatibility with Environment (EMVU).

Chapter 6 - Important Tips on the Treatment

The Treatment Is Over - Keep Moving!

After completing the course of cancer treatment, I still practice my Nordic walking, preferably every day but at least five times a week. Every time I cover some 3 to 4 kilometers in half an hour.

Over a week that makes about 20 km, which burns around 2,000 kcal – outdoors, in the fresh air! My dear wife often accompanies me, and we enjoy working out together.

As far as the speed is concerned, we usually try to walk fast, but at a comfortable pace, without exertion. One the other hand, if you walk slowly and without effort, you won't achieve anything – in this case, fitness will remain your pipe dream.
At the same time, walking too fast, close to jogging, with puffing and sweating, is all the more useless.

If you want to learn more about this subject, I would highly recommend you read the book "Forever Young" (see Bibliography) by the "fitness guru" Dr. med. Ulrich Th. Strunz. My recommendation is as follows: after you are cured of cancer, find your sport and keep moving!

By the way, in summer we try to have breakfast only after our morning walk, since exercising is more effective on an empty stomach: with carbohydrates being depleted in the morning, our body burns more fat and builds up more muscles. More details can be found in the book "Forever Young" (see Bibliography).

However, in winter we usually do Nordic walking during our lunch break, simply because it is often too cold early in the morning before breakfast.

Chapter 6 - Important Tips on the Treatment

A good route...

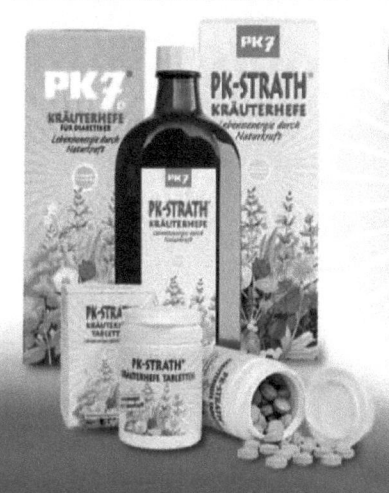

STRATH

Strath-Labor GmbH
93093 Donaustauf
Phone 09403/9509-0
strath-labor@t-online.de
www.strath-labor.de

...To improve health!

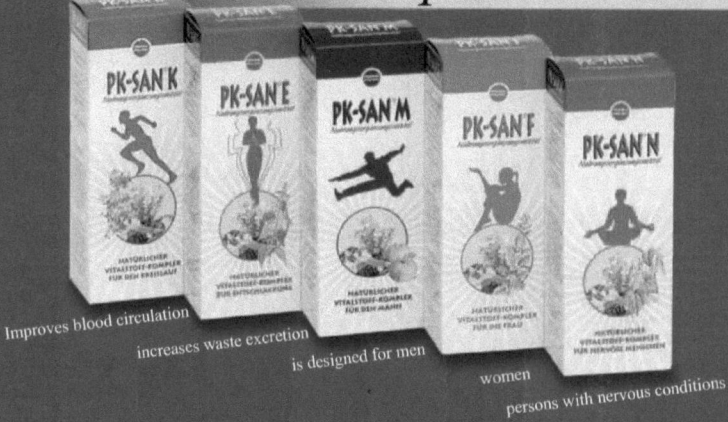

Improves blood circulation
increases waste excretion
is designed for men
women
persons with nervous conditions

- Natural ingredients, no artificial additives
- Vitamins, minerals, protein, enzymes – derived from fruits, vegetables, herbs and yeast.

Chapter 6 - Important Tips on the Treatment

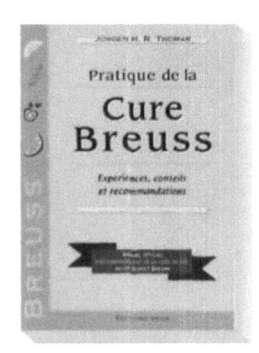

Jürgen H.R. Thomar
Practicing the Breuss Treatment
Experience, advice and recommendations
User guide to the Rudolf Breuss juice treatment
VEGA Publishing House, 19, rue Saint-Severin, Paris 750005
2007, translation and adaptation from German by Peter Schmidt
This is the French edition of my book on cancer treatment.
A5, 176 pages, paperback
€ (France/Germany/Austria) 13.00
ISBN 978-2-85829-470-4

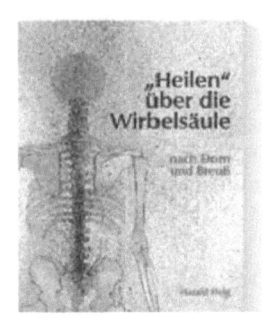

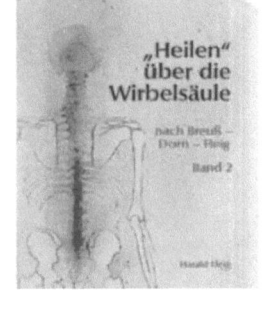

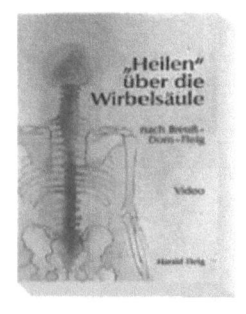

Harald Fleig

„Healing the Spinal Column After Dorn and Breuss"

Volume 1

The Breuss massage is a gentle, energetic back massage which dissolves mental and physical tension according to the theory which treats intervertebral discs not as being "rubbed off", but "degenerated", and assumes that they can be completely regenerated.

A5, 96 pages, paperback
€(Germany/Austria/Switzerland) 9.20
ISBN 3-98051382-0-7

Harald Fleig

„Healing the Spinal Column After Dorn and Breuss"

Volume 2

This volume by Harald Fleig provides a detailed and comprehensible description of other data and experience received from practicing the Breuss and Dorn method. At the same time, he points out various mistakes made during application of the Breuss and Dorn method by other therapists.
A5, 336 pages, paperback
€(Germany/Austria/Switzerland) 15.00
ISBN 3-9805138-1-5

Harald Fleig

„Healing the Spinal Column After Dorn and Breuss"

DVD

This DVD provides a clear and comprehensible overview of both therapies – the Breuss massage and the Dorn therapy.
The DVD is an ideal complement to seminars conducted by the training center of Brigitte and Harald Fleig in Wehr (Baden, Germany).

DVD, runtime: approx. 120 minutes,
€(Germany/Austria/Switzerland) 20.00

CHAPTER 7
Strengthening Your Immune System

⌘

Factors that Weaken Our Immune System

In this Chapter I would like to give the floor to Dr. Veronica Carstens, MD. The fact is that if we want to be healthy and to stay that way, we cannot do it without a strong immune system.

In her scientific paper "Empirical cancer diagnosis and therapy" she, in particular, says, *"Cancer is a disease which takes many years before becoming evident. Cancer is said to be caused by a variety of reasons, but it certainly can be targeted, at least, in some spheres. However, without changing our life habits we still face the danger of further negative impact produced by a number of harmful habits. What are these factors?"*

Dr. Carstens goes on to say, *"Cancer researchers constantly point out the following factors:*

- *Constitutional weakness, i.e., inherited predisposition,*
- *unbalanced diet, and*
- *emotional stress".*

She goes on to write, *"Johannes Kuhl, a well-known doctor and naturalist, states that the following three reasons lead to acid-alkaline imbalance and thereby to severe cellular malfunction.*

Chapter 7 - Strengthening Your Immune System

There appears a damaged cell which is not cancerous yet. If it is continuously affected by aggravating factors, it eventually becomes cancerous. These aggravating factors include:

- *oxygen deficiency (lack of exercise in the open air),*

- *chemical substances the body derives from air, water, food and medication,*

- *radiation from X-rays, building materials and tentatively – so-called ground radiation* (to these, I'd add electric smog, mobile phones, TV screens, etc.),

- *viral infections,*

- *hidden sites of inflammation (for example, teeth and tonsils),*

- *dental amalgam fillings, and*

- *infections caused by yeast fungus Candida* [11]

The citations above are taken from a paper by Dr. Veronica Carstens, MD, the wife of our former Federal President.

---

11) Yeast fungus Candida is a natural inhabitant of the intestines which gets along quite well with good intestinal bacteria; it is regulated by microorganisms. If the intestines contain "bad" bacteria, the fungus can grow unrestricted. The diet oversaturated with yeasts, sugar and dairy products can exacerbate the problem by contributing to fast development of Candida. It damages the intestines and causes serious symptoms and associated diseases.
Overuse of antibiotics, cortisone treatment, excessive sugar, unbalanced diet, hormonal contraceptives or heavy metals can trigger the growth of yeast fungi and eventually cause enterobrosia. It can result in intestinal particles entering the blood instead of escaping through defecation. The immune system gets overloaded with foreign substances, which leads to allergies, etc.
When Candida starts growing, the patient feels drawn to those products which feed the fungus. For example, sweets, white yeast bread, dairy products, alcohol.

Chapter 7 - Strengthening Your Immune System

Factors that Strengthen Our Immune System

Let me once again quote Dr. Carstens here, as her statements reveal the basis of both the fasting therapy by Breuss and his success in naturopathy.

Dr. Carstens writes, *"Some of these factors can be discovered only by a doctor, for instance, a hidden site of inflammation, viral infection or deleterious effect from amalgam and Candida.*

Other aggravating factors mostly depend on a patient. So we are anything but powerless against cancer! While being healthy, we can try to adopt a balanced lifestyle and prevent cancer. It does not mean depriving ourselves of the joy of life or giving up the pursuit of happiness. On the contrary, we'll feel stronger, livelier and happier.

But when diagnosed with cancer, we can significantly aid recovery through our behavior. And the simplest path to recovery runs through **nutrition***. In this case, we talk of eating plain natural food that is not chemically treated, canned or overcooked.*

If you are not able to eat raw fruits and vegetables, they can be slightly stewed.

In the morning it is especially useful to drink a glass of vegetable mixture – half glass of carrot juice and half glass of beet juice, homemade with a squeezer or ready-made bottled juice (health food store). The well-known Breuss vegetable juice is also very useful - it can be purchased in the same store or pharmacy.

Sugar, white flour and the products containing them, such as white bread, buns, pastry and noodles must be avoided. They are useless food. Besides, sugar and starch in their composition are sources of high lactic acid in cancer cells, as well as fuel sources for Candida".

Chapter 7 - Strengthening Your Immune System

Dr. Carstens goes on to say, *"And finally, take a look at yet another observation. Just like the growth rate of newborn humans and newborn animals of various species depends on protein content in breast milk, the tumor growth rate depends on protein content in food. It means that*

The rate of growth of the tumor, whether fast or slow, depends on the cancer patient!

If the patient follows a low-protein diet, the tumor cannot develop as in order to grow it needs protein. On the other hand, protein deficiency causes the body to split protein in locations where it is not crucial for survival, i.e., in tumor.

These facts lead inevitably to the conclusion that during post-surgery and expected recurrence period (let me explain: the reason for the latter is often an incomplete excision of a tumor, which in a while later can lead to recurrence of the disease) *protein intake is to be sharply reduced"*.

The citation above is also taken from the paper by Dr. Veronica Carstens, MD.

Does Protein Cause Hyperacidity?

Acid-Alkaline Balance

The acid-alkaline balance has a significant impact on human health. The acid-alkaline ratio is determined by measuring pH levels on a scale of 0 ("acid") to 14 ("alkaline"). If the correlation of acids and alkali is 50:50, the solution has a pH of 7.0, which is a neutral reaction. However, the correlation of acids and alkali in our body is not 50:50. Research shows that between 80% and 90% of Germans has a permanent tendency to slight hyperacidity. What are the reasons and consequences of this phenomenon?

Is Malnutrition to Blame?

First and foremost, the main reason is considered to be an unbalanced diet. For most people, it primarily contains acid forming products, such as meat, fast food, white flour, sugar, coffee, carbonated drinks and alcohol. And only 20% of the food consumed is made up of alkaline forming products, for example, fruits, vegetables and natural table or mineral water; their share is often even lower than that. With this in mind, it is crucial not to be misled by the popular belief that hyperacidity is caused by products with acid taste – and to remember that it is only caused by products that are "metabolised" into acid in the process of digestion. Thus, foods high in sugar can cause hyperacidity, while vinegar, on the contrary, increases alkaline levels.

But our daily diet is not the only factor involved. Stress and emotional have an effect the acid-base balance too. Irritation, overload, disappointments, fear, noise and nicotine also cause hyperacidity, as do environmental toxins and medications.

Chapter 7 - Strengthening Your Immune System

If hyperacidity progresses, then such symptoms may appear as chronic apathy towards all things exterior, fast fatigability, susceptibility to infection, a depressed mood, anxiety, muscle spasms, joint problems. Hair loss and eczema can even be extreme manifestations of hyperacidity.

In such cases, people usually say they feel washed-out *(pun on the German word ausgelaugt which means 1) washed-out, worn-out, and 2) salt washed, leached).* If the body does not restore its mineral balance, it will have to use its own mineral resources. And doing nothing about it can result in such serious diseases like gout, kidney stones, rheumatism, diabetes or even myocardial infarction (heart attack) and cancer.

Testing Your pH Levels

You should know better than go to such extremes. The easiest way to find out if you are acidic is to use uric acid test strips from the pharmacy. The thing is that excess acid is removed through the kidneys and it can be detected in urine. For this test, immediately after getting up in the morning you need to dip the test strip (for example, Merck pH Indicator Strips Neutralit) in urine for a short time – the color will change. Compare the result (color) with the color of the pH on the test strip box.

The acidity level constantly changes during the day, so it is better to measure it in the morning. Neutral urine acidity is the best result (professional jargon has it as "pH 7"). If the indicator is below 7, it is said to be acid urine, in case it is above 7, the urine is alkaline. Values within the range of 6.5 to 7.5 are considered to be normal.

Chapter 7 - Strengthening Your Immune System

Conclusions Based on Test Results

If your indicators show hyperacidity, you need to

- firstly, reconsider your eating habits. As the human body (its solid components) consists of 80% alkaline forming and 20% acid forming substances, a whole 80 years ago dietitians recommended that we stick to the same ratio in our daily diet (that is, 80% of the diet should consist of fruits and vegetables!),
- try to drink a sufficient amount of carbon-free water

- follow the advice of Breuss and exercise outdoors for an hour every day, also because sports help the body excrete acid through sweating.

Less Protein means More Health?

Let me once again draw your attention to the paper by Dr. Carstens. She writes the following on this issue,: *"It is a well-known fact that many chronic patients have tissue hyperacidity. It is caused by both abovementioned carbohydrates (sugar and starch) and, first and foremost, by protein (according to F.F. Zander "Acid-base equilibrium in humans", Hippokrates, Stuttgart, 1953).*

What are the risks caused by hyperacidity?

- *The cellular respiration level is reduced (as excessive H-ions bind oxygen).*

- *Uric acid is poorly excreted from the body and its high levels may cause salt crystals to deposit in the body's tissues.*

- *An acid environment encourages the growth of microorganisms.*

That leads to frequent urinary tract infections, which weaken a human being."

Beware of a High-Protein Diet Leading to Hyperacidity!

Dr. Carstens goes on to say, *"To reduce hyperacidity (or prevent it), you need to reduce your protein intake, simultaneously increasing the share of fruits, vegetables and salads in your diet* (my note: not only fruits and salads, but also tasty and healthy slices of vegetables should be eaten raw as much as possible!)

Thus, tissue hyperacidity is a negative consequence of eating too much high-protein food. There is also another danger: protein is deposited on the arterial walls, which leads to oxygen depletion of tissues and their disfunction (Prof. Vendt "Protein storage disorders", Haug, Heidelberg, 1984).

Another risk of consuming excessive protein is dangerous putrefaction products in the intestines caused by bacterial decomposition.

This danger is caused by two factors:

1.   It has been proved that a regular correlation exists between intestinal flora and the level of white blood cells and blood pigment.
2.   The consequences are further oxygen depletion (as red blood pigment serves as an oxygen carrier in blood) and weaken endogenous defense resulting from the reduction in white blood cells."

The citations above are taken from the paper by Dr. Carstens entitled "Empirical cancer diagnosis and therapy", which quickly disappeared from bookstore shelves and, unfortunately, hasn't been republished since. Thank God I have a copy of this paper.

Chapter 7 - Strengthening Your Immune System

To sum up everything stated above, I offer a conclusion which can be viewed as a recommendation:

The decision on how long (if at all) one's immune system will keep cancer at bay is actually a personal one made by a healthy person!

〰〰

For the post-treatment period:

Tips for Healthy Eating

Lessons Learned from Fasting Therapy

The Breuss fasting therapy can – or, even better, must – serve as an impulse for lifestyle changes.

The positive experience obtained during fasting often leads to the development of a more conscientious attitude to your own health and rethinking your lifestyle. In our hurly-burly times, fasting is a kind of re-evaluation, taking an inward turn. It helps people to stabilize their inner balance and contains considerable potential for spiritual and intellectual enrichment.

The Cure, or Fasting Therapy, by Rudolf Breuss can become the beginning of purposeful and useful weight reduction. The reason is that maintaining a reasonably limited diet, chewing food more slowly and doing regular exercise (for instance, Nordic Walking or long distance walking) not only contribute to successful treatment, but also turn out to be important health-enhancing factors.

The Importance of a Fully Functional Metabolism

Our body is shaped by what we eat and drink. Each tiny individual cell needs special nutrition to perform its functions in the body. For these nutrients to get to the right place, a fully functional metabolism is of utmost importance.

In its turn, a healthy metabolism requires healthy intestines which work on processing our food. The Breuss fasting

Chapter 7 - Strengthening Your Immune System

therapy will help to lay the foundation for such healthy intestines.

However, if you want to improve your health on a long-term basis, it is absolutely vital to change your long-term eating habits.

Don't Eat in Haste!

This refers to both conscious selection of food products (fresh and natural) and eating them "properly".

In this respect, chewing food slowly and thoroughly is especially **important**. Firstly, it trains the sense of taste and, secondly, it substantially unloads the digestive tract, and last, but not least, you will feel full faster. The thing is that a sense of fullness usually comes only 20 minutes after eating.

Those who ignore this tip and swallow food in haste, in a rush, frequently overeat. No wonder this eating habit is often accompanied by obesity, digestive problems, gastric ulcer and other unpleasant things.

Stay Healthy as Long as Possible

If you want to stay healthy after the treatment course, consider the recommendation to eat plain natural food, that is not chemically treated, canned or overcooked products and, in any case, not reheated food.

Also, do not use any readymade food, ready-to-cook products from supermarket refrigerated display cases - all products must be as fresh as possible!

Chapter 7 - Strengthening Your Immune System

You don't have to follow these recommendations one hundred percent, even ninety percent would be quite enough!

If you are not able to eat raw fruits and vegetables, they can be slightly stewed. **Note**! The abovementioned "not able to eat raw fruits and vegetables" means that they should be eaten raw if possible. Set two or three "vegetable days" a week when you'll have only fruits and vegetables on your menu. As you see, your way of eating is being gradually changed!

If you don't eat yet eat just fruits for breakfast, as we do, you will need the tips below to make the transition to healthy morning eating.

> **Tip #1:** *in the morning it is especially healthy to drink a glass of vegetable mixture – half a glass of carrot juice and half a glass of beet juice, homemade or readymade.*

and

> **Tip #2:** *it is also very healthy to drink a homemade glass of Breuss vegetable juice, which you got to know during treatment.*

We All Have the Power to Reduce the Risk of Cancer

On the occasion of World Cancer Day, February 4, 2010, German Cancer Aid and the Union for International Cancer Control (UICC, Union Internationale Contre le Cancer) drew everyone's attention to the fact that a conscientious attitude to one's own health can prevent cancer. Prof. Dr. Med. Harald zur Hausen, the German Cancer Aid's President, stresses that *"We all have the power to reduce cancer risk. Long-term changes in lifestyle can prevent almost half of all cancers."*

Chapter 7 - Strengthening Your Immune System

Those who develop a conscientious attitude to their health when young, have a good chance of living a long and healthy life. For middle-aged people, too, it is not too late to adopt the following rules, in particular, aimed at lowering cancer risk:

- exercise in the open air,
- eat healthy food,
- avoid putting on weight,
- give up smoking,
- be careful with UV exposure,
- reduce alcohol consumption; and
- protect yourself from cancer-associated infections.

In order to encourage people to reconsider their lifestyle, German Cancer Aid addresses parents and grandparents, urging them to be role models for their children and grandchildren. Dr. Zur Hausen says *"Lifestyle plays a vital role in keeping you and your descendants healthy. Those who run unreasonable health risks damage the quality of their own life and that of their children. Help us make healthy living a norm for everybody."*

I've got nothing to add here.

What Must Be Avoided by All Means

Now I deliberately want to reiterate that sugar, white flour and the products containing them, such as white bread, buns (even whole-grain ones!), pastry and noodles, must be avoided (see References, Appendix 6, "Sugar? No, thank you!"). They are useless. Besides, sugar and starch in their composition are sources of high lactic acid in cancer cells, as well as fuel sources for Candida (see the chapters above).

Besides, pork must be avoided in any form, no matter whether it is pork chop or sausage. It stands to reason that eating pork is strongly prohibited in Islamic countries, and even in colder regions. And what about this country? If you've seen hormonally-doped pigs on huge breeding farms just once, you know what I mean.

Reheated Food

R. Breuss says that when a person feels hungry, it is a sign of death of the cells which have to be replaced by eating a portion of food. In case of eating reheated food poor in vitamins, these cells will not be replaced in the long-term.

Reheated food is, therefore, worthless and in certain circumstances even dangerous. It is nothing but useless food (ballast), hardly considered food anymore.

The term *food* should apply only to the products which sustain life *(pun on the German word Lebensmittel (food products), the literal meaning of which is "a means of life")*.

It is important to know that precooked fast-frozen food is also considered reheated food.

Protein Revisited

According to Dr. Carstens, protein is crucial for nourishing both cancer patients and cancer survivors. That's why she gives the following advice on protein intake:

Chapter 7 - Strengthening Your Immune System

- During the first 3-4 months after cancer surgery (this also refers to chemotherapy, and most certainly to the post-treatment period following the Breuss Cure, only for a shorter time), the eating of "any animal products" (except for butter and cream) is not allowed. This means that dairy products and eggs are not allowed either.

- After that, it is absolutely forbidden to eat "dead animal products", that is meat, fish, poultry, with an exception made for small amounts of milk, cheese and eggs.

- At later stages, when health in general and the immune system in particular stabilize, the reduced consumption of meat is recommended (perhaps once or maximum twice a week), but absolutely no pork!

While maintaining the strict protein-poor diet mentioned above (which is easy to remember due to its figurative name "no animal products"), one shouldn't fear that a lack of protein can have a negative impact on the body; consider the data which is not commonly known but undoubtedly true:

- whole-wheat bran bread contains   14% protein
- meat contains   20% protein
- soy contains   40% protein
- hard cheese contains   45% protein

After the Breuss treatment, the necessary protein is provided by bran bread, muesli, as well as by adding small amounts of soy to food. However, consuming the products above will not lead to protein overload accompanied by the unpleasant consequences mentioned above.

Healthy Food

Eating healthy food depends entirely on your willingness, and nothing but your willingness.

Eating healthy food depends entirely on your willingness, and nothing but your willingness.

If I have only succeeded in having you:

- be more careful when reading labels with ingredients when shopping next time,
- put back on the shelf any "beautifully and brightly" packaged product,
- fill your shopping cart with more useful products instead,

I will have achieved a lot.
And on behalf of *your* body, I say

THANK YOU!

Chapter 7 - Strengthening Your Immune System

Tips on Drinking "Good Water"

"There's no healing without water!"
(Johann Wolfgang von Goethe, "Faust")

Crystal-clear spring water scooped up in wonderful nature's lap amid fresh wildwood – is there anything healthier in the world?

Unfortunately, now it has become nothing but a dream...

Having faith in this dream and reading newspaper articles claiming that tap water is constantly under control which makes its quality perfect, many people will probably say:

*"There´s nothing **better than tap** water. That's because this water is the most regulated foodstuff in Germany!"*

Tap Water:
the Most Regulated Foodstuff (?)

Water for drinking and cooking comes mainly from a tap in and out apartment. That's where the trouble lies. We certainly do read in newspapers that recent water tests prove the high quality of tap water, and that the health limits for hazardous substances are not exceeded, thereby concluding that tap water quality complies with the standards enforced by law.

However, some issues are withheld by newspapers, namely, the fact that more than once, over the last 20 years, the maximum contaminant levels for hazardous substances have

Chapter 7 - Strengthening Your Immune System

been dramatically and significantly increased. Otherwise, water would no more comply with the previously established maximum contaminant levels for hazardous substances. This means no efforts have been made to at least protect water quality from deteriorating, instead the authorities opt for lower quality standards.

Figuratively speaking, 20 years ago the tap water we consume today would have been recycled as hazardous waste.

Such policy is, probably, accounted for by economic considerations, as the implementation of new advanced methods of water purification from increasingly extensive bacterial, hormonal and drug pollution would cost many millions and billions Euro more.

Those who, like me, live in the countryside, can often, even nowadays, see villagers vigorously spreading manure over their fields. The fact that by doing this they not only poison the soil to be inherited by their children and grandchildren, but also increasingly pollute our drinking water with salts, does not obviously trouble them - nor does it trouble the State. For "they have fresh countryside air here". Someone likes it... I don't though.

If drinking water contains nitrate concentration of 30 mg/liter, as we have here, this water cannot actually be used for drinking. Besides, it should be taken into account that water samples for checking maximum contaminant levels for hazardous substances, that is for water quality tests, are collected not in our homes, but whole kilometers away from them, near the "source", which is the water supply plant. The water-pipe contaminating effect, including that of water supply pipes in our houses (lead and copper pipes, bacteria etc.), is not taken into consideration. Moreover, the tests do not cover a whole range of contaminants. <u>For instance, they do not take into account traces of medications, such as hormones, antibiotics or analgesics.</u>

Various indicators of maximum contaminant levels are just unreasonably high. For example, according to the German Drinking Water Regulations, since 2003 the copper indicator has been increased to 2.0 mg/liter, while the EU recommendations on water for infants set the limit for copper indicator at 0.1 mg/liter, which means that the German norm is 20 times higher! The lead limit is now 25 micrograms, which is too high, though by 2013 it is to be reduced to 10 micrograms in three stages (the question is why it takes <u>so long</u> and why the target limit is not <u>much lower</u> <u>than that</u>).

Only after all tests at the water supply plant, does this "elixir of life" (in the current context this epithet sounds almost anachronistic) make its long way to our homes through water pipes tens and sometimes hundreds years old. Then water goes through the indoor plumbing system - not always new - and eventually comes to our taps, releasing something we are still trustfully calling "water, drinking water".

Thus, there are big, even gigantic differences between dream and reality, between crystal-clear, transparent, fresh and healthy water and the liquid released by our water taps.

What about harmful substances in drinking water in the place where you live? What about the pollution of <u>your</u> drinking water with harmful substances? I'm sure they exist in your water, too. Such substances as nitrates, lead, pesticides are found in drinking water even if the maximum contaminant levels are under strict control, a fact which is well recognized by the water supply plant authorities.

Each of us should investigate the situation with harmful substances in water at the local water supply plant. Usually, these are 35 different substances, including lead, chlorine and nitrates. Ask if the water-supply plant laboratory checks the water for bacteria, viruses, fungi, hormones, analgesics, medications, etc. These questions are not usually asked. That's why nothing is done.

World Water Quality Assessment

Within the framework of one of the UN projects, its experts issued a report on the situation with world water, the so-called World Water Development Report, in which they compared the quality of water in 122 countries.

Finland topped the list with an indicator +1.85. The worst situation is in Belgium with an indicator of -2.25. The report states that the reasons include the poor condition of ground waters, high level of industrial sewage waters pollution and the under-treatment of water. Thus, the country where the headquarters of many EU institutions and located and the country where provides the world with the well-known mineral waters Spa and Chaudfontaine, found itself below India, Jordan and nine African countries that keep the European outsider company at the bottom of the list.

While drawing their charts, the European experts took into account not only the purity of rivers and ground waters, but also the willingness of the country to improve the quality of its water supply. And here again Belgium will have to make up for lost time, as in 2000 the Kingdom received a warning from the EU Court of Justice concerning the lack of fully functional purification facilities in the Brussels region. However, even today much of the water polluted by the population of over one million people is still flowing as muddy slush to the small River Senne embedded in concrete.

Germany found itself <u>second</u> to last <u>among EU countries</u> and in the middle of the general list with **a negative indicator of −0.06.** Germany, in the study, was in one position above Zimbabwe and five positions <u>below</u> Botswana.

(from Spiegel ONLINE, March 5, 2003).

So, Can We Drink Tap Water?

For me and for us, that's out of the question.

Is Mineral Water the Best Quality Water?

As many people have also realized what is happening to our tap water, they say:

*"I only drink **mineral water** for it is top quality! And it has so many minerals!"*

Is that so?

In 2000, GEO magazine published an article on the situation with drinking water in Germany entitled "Drinking water as a man-made product". This article states among other things: "….However, neither mineral nor table water is absolutely pure. It is often impossible to drink - at least because of its taste - without further additional treatment. This means artificially removing different undesirable substances (for example, iron) from water…"

As regards well-praised minerals contained in mineral water, Ingo Froböse, a Sports Science expert, states the following, "Every person of normal nutrition satisfies the need for minerals mainly through the consumption of solid food".

The question as to whether the human body is generally able to process mineral substances contained in mineral water is a controversial one. "In mineral water minerals are present as molecules, which are too big to be digested by the body." Froböse states that these substances are excreted in the urine unchanged. In this respect mineral water is no better than tap water which contains minerals as well.

At the same time, we have approached the stopping point beyond which I would rather not go, confining myself instead to a few comments on mineral water with carbon

Chapter 7 - Strengthening Your Immune System

dioxide (no matter whether it is called "heavy carbonated" or "medium carbonated" water), as well as on the bottles it is sold in. Carbonated mineral water makes your body even more acidic. **Avoid acidification** (read more at the beginning of this chapter) **and drink decarbonated (still) water as it does not contain carbon dioxide.**

Close attention should be paid to **nitrite and nitrate levels in water.** Naturally- occurring nitrates do not represent a health threat. Due to gut bacteria or long-term storage of food, nitrate (NO_3^-) can turn into nitrite (NO_2^-). And nitrite is a substance of concern.

Nitrite can get into the body directly from vegetables or salt-cured meat products. However, most nitrites enter our body as a result of oral bacteria converting nitrate to nitrite (so-called nitrate reduction).

Some 70%-80% of nitrates get into the human body from vegetables each day. Depending on local conditions, nitrates contained in drinking water can be a serious additional burden on the body.

Nitrates are excreted primarily by the urinary system. Approximately 6% of nitrates are converted by saliva to nitrites, which in their turn enter other biological liquids, such as digestive juice and urine. Thus, the nitrite level in saliva directly correlates with the amount of nitrate consumed.

Nitrite is a health hazard for infants in the early months of life (cyanochroia, cyanosis), as it prevents oxygen delivery to the blood. These risks are mainly related to drinking water with high nitrate levels. It is best to use water suitable for baby food production or water with no nitrites or nitrates (this should be indicated on the label).

And you should always drink water from glass bottles as health experts state that plasticizers of plastic bottles migrate to water. In their opinion, the softer the plastic, the more dangerous it is.

Meanwhile, some people say, *"I drink only clear, devoid of any harmful substances,* **distilled water** *– for me it is the best water. In the USA* **distilled water** *has been consumed by millions of people for years!"*

Distilled Water

Aqua Destillata (Distilled Water) - to Drink Or Not to Drink?

Distilled water is obtained through distillation (evaporation with consequent condensation) from tap water or previously purified water.

Distilled water has for decades been considered and is still considered by many doctors and scientists as unsuitable for drinking as it can cause cells to "rupture" or lead to "gastric hemorrhage".

However, today we often hear exactly the opposite; for example, followers of the Fit-for-Life (USA) claim that what is good for accumulators cannot be bad for humans. **Their most important argument is that all harmful substances are removed.**

The Fit-for-Life (USA)'s followers state that distilled water does not pose a threat as it used to be believed, a fact supported by many absolutely healthy people. Distilled water is now more and more often being promoted as healthy. It is totally stripped of substances like calcium, which in due time can cause deposits (fear-inducing calcinosis) in blood vessels.

It was believed, especially in Germany, that as distilled water is completely stripped of minerals, endogenous cells try to level the difference in dissolved particles concentration from both sides, which fills them with water to the extent that they simply rupture. However, water completely stripped of minerals and salts does not get into cells because these important substances also enter the body through solid food and mix in the stomach.

But here comes another dissenting opinion: being completely stripped of minerals, distilled water leaches **important** natural organic substances vital for the body. What is my opinion on distilled water? Am I convinced by numerous arguments claiming that it is "good"?

Taking into account the fact that the debate on distilled water in Germany is still not over, I wouldn't give any advice either for or against it.

What Water do the Thomars Drink?

In any case we never drink:

- tap,
- mineral,
- distilled water.

My wife and I prefer water made at our home with the help of advanced **filtration technologies**.

All the details are given below:

Water Purification Filters

Reverse osmosis[12] is something that you can't do without! What filtration technologies are used nowadays? There is a wide choice, ranging from cheap countertop water filters and water filter jugs to electronic carbonation devices (Wassersprudler) and similar equipment. Prices range from 20 to 900 euros. So, what is the effect?

Some devices only add carbon dioxide to unpurified tap water, others with the help of cation exchange only remove calcium and magnesium from drinking water.

Filtered substances are replaced by other cations. It results in decreasing the water's pH level to 4 (while the optimal level would be 6.8). This leads to acidification of the body (Note! Acidification threat again, read more at the beginning of the chapter). Other substances are, as a rule, not filtered. Besides, these filters are favorable environment for the growth of microorganisms because of stale water. Thus, they do not solve our problem!

So what shall we choose? Experts say that if you want to drink clean healthy water, you cannot do without reverse osmosis technologies. We installed such a device three years ago.

---

12) Reverse osmosis is a physical water treatment process. It is used for purifying drinking, industrial and aquarium water, as well as treating sewage water. The same principle is used for producing fruit juice concentrates. Reverse osmosis uses pressure to overcome natural osmosis. The pressure applied should be higher than osmotic pressure which tends to level the solute concentration. Osmotic pressure of drinking water is below 2 bars, the pressure applied for reverse osmosis constitutes 4 to 30 bars, depending on the membrane used and unit configuration

("Wikipedia")

Chapter 7 - Strengthening Your Immune System

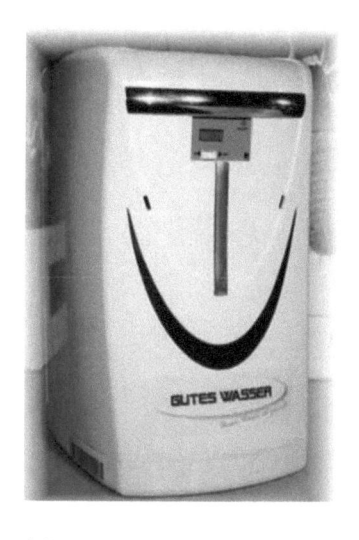

It supplies us with healthy soft water from a separate tap and removes almost all harmful substances from the water we drink. Undoubtedly, there are various devices present on the market. You can choose anything you want. It is **important** to select the one that uses the **reverse osmosis system with a high-efficiency filter**

The "smiling device" above (it seems to be smiling, doesn't it?) is called simply "**Good Water**" (Germ. Gutes Wasser). This name is taken from my book "**Rudolf Breuss Fasting Therapy – Simply Ingenious**" and related to the story of Dr. P. (see Chapter 1 of the book).

Purpose And Mechanism of Reverse Osmosis

Osmosis is based on the natural process through which plants, for example, absorb moisture from soil with their root cells. A similar process takes place in the human body during metabolic processes across cell membranes. If two different liquids are separated by a semipermeable membrane, liquid molecules will, according to the principle of Brownian motion of molecules, start moving toward a more concentrated solute. This creates osmotic pressure. To obtain the best purified water, significantly higher pressure is exerted on the high concentration side. Thus, the process is reversed, causing what is called "reverse osmosis".

Cleaning Water with Advanced Filtration Technology

The "heart" of this system is a multilayer filter membrane with holes so tiny as to admit only water molecules. Thus, the membrane purifies our tap water from heavy metals, bacteria and viruses.

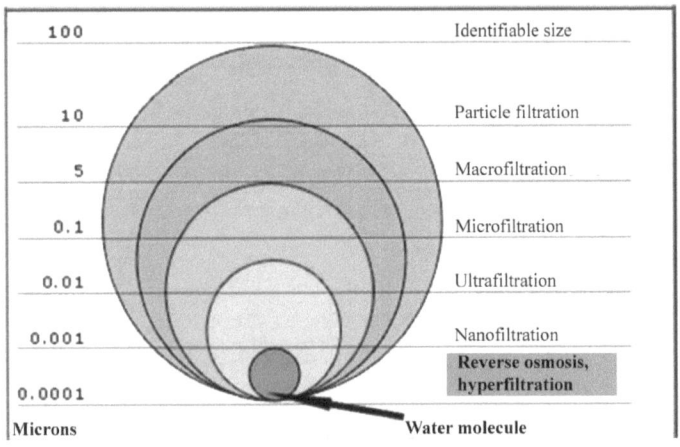

Microns	
100	Identifiable size
10	Particle filtration
5	Macrofiltration
0.1	Microfiltration
0.01	Ultrafiltration
0.001	Nanofiltration
0.0001	Reverse osmosis, hyperfiltration
	Water molecule

Comparison of dimensions

The external diameter of 100 microns equates approximately to a hair's breadth. Filtered water can, in terms of its purity, be compared to several natural sources.

Advantages of Such Equipment

What are the advantages of a device like this? Here they are:

• the cleanest, soft, tasty and refreshing tap water for drinking and cooking which makes tea and coffee, as well as vegetables and soups healthier and more delicious! This water can be used even for washing hair: with it, your hair is more shiny and manageable, and is easier to dye (as the water is softer and purified from chemicals and harmful substances).

Chapter 7 - Strengthening Your Immune System

- A reasonable price, which means minimal expenses for producing drinking water.

- No need to transport and store drinking water bottles or to recycle the containers.

- And the most important thing: this unit filters out **harmful substances** contained in water. We have maximum contaminant levels for some really harmful and dangerous substances!

- It means that these substances can be present in our drinking water on "absolutely official" grounds

Remember the following: in the Global Drinking Water Quality Rating, Germany occupies the second to last position among EU countries, and it finds itself below such countries as Ghana, Bangladesh, Turkey, Bulgaria, Jamaica and Ecuador!

What's in Our Drinking Water?

Our – and your – tap water contains poisonous substances listed below:

- aluminum,
- arsenic,
- asbestos,
- bacteria,
- benzene,
- lead
- chlorine
- DDT,

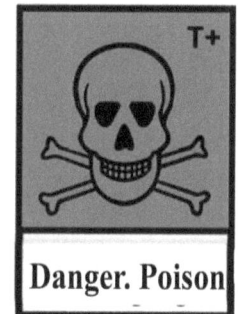

Chapter 7 - Strengthening Your Immune System

- fluorides
- herbicides,
- lime,
- copper,
- nitrates,
- PAH (polycyclic aromatic hydrocarbons),
- pentachlorophenol,
- pesticides,
- fungi,
- mercury,
- strontium,
- toluene,
- uranium,
- viruses and
- xylene.

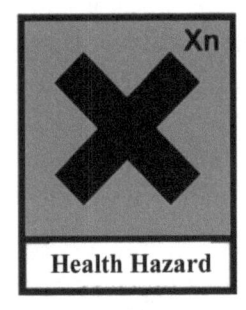

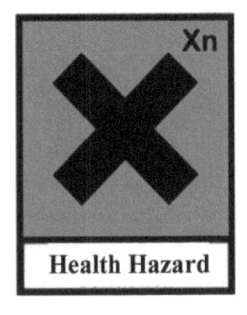

There are maximum contaminant levels for these poisons, which, are constantly increased (as they have to), otherwise these health limits would be constantly violated and water couldn't be used for drinking!

It's fuzzy logic, you will say. Instead of increasing maximum contaminant levels, it would be more reasonable to make sure these poisons do not get into water.

But "Good water" unit filters out 99% of these substances, including hormones and medications!

Chapter 7 - Strengthening Your Immune System

The result is almost 100% clean water
- transparent,
- soft, and
- healthy!

Now I bet you want to know where you can order this "Good water" unit and find out its price. To find it out, you just need to consult the Index in the appendix.

So, What Is "Good Water"?

Let's summarize everything said on "good water":

- the less carbon in the water, the better it is,
- natural spring water is surely the best choice,
- running water through a reverse osmosis system repeatedly produces the result closest to this natural spring water.

If by sharing my perspectives on the issue of good water I succeeded in having you:

- start active research on healthy, good water,
- as a result, substitute carbonated mineral water with decarbonated mineral water,

I would achieve a lot for your body. Wouldn't I?

Mothballs, Water Veins and Earth Radiation

Consider another group of factors that can also bolster or weaken your immune system.

Mothballs

If you have naphthalene, camphor (synthetic camphor

Chapter 7 - Strengthening Your Immune System

obtained from waste coal at gas plants), DDT or similar poisons to keep away moths and cockroaches, or fly sprays, air fresheners in the bathroom, etc., you should be able to get rid of all these poisons. And afterwards for 14 days running (once a day, but do it properly), burn fragrant resin as incense (for example, Weihrauch, a resin collected by ants, stored in and obtained from ant hills; can be purchased in pharmacies and beauty stores). Breuss is absolutely clear on this: if you have the abovementioned poisons in you apartment, you will probably not be able to cure the disease – that is how dangerous they are. Instead of using naphthalene, synthetic camphor, DDT, etc., it is much healthier to use natural materials. For example, lavender, walnut leaves, hops, woodruff, wormwood, plant extracts soap, curd soap, tobacco, perfume or natural camphor produced from wood shavings of the camphor tree.

Water Veins and Earth Radiation

According to Breuss's experience, most patients lie on top of so-called "damaging earth rays" which are even more dangerous when they cross. That is why, as a preventive measure, it is desirable to consult a "dowser" or a "commuter" to detect these dangerous places in your house, and to make sure that your bed is in a safe place. There are people who do not believe this, but if you consult three dowsers and each finds water veins in the same spot, then they can't be totally wrong. My wife and I invited such experts to examine our bedroom and they detected a geopathogenic zone under my bed. We moved our beds half a meter aside and are now sleeping in a safe area.

Please see the appendix for the addresses of such experts.

Chapter 7 - Strengthening Your Immune System

GOOD WATER

Our water is healthy!

Unfortunately, our attitude today to water as cure and food No. 1 is rather irresponsible. It is hard to imagine how many hazardous substances our tap water contains: heavy metals, hormones, analgesics, etc.!

Ask someone at your water supply plant what hazardous substances they test water for (note that they do not test it for most hazards, nor do they test it for hormones, bacteria, viruses and medications found in ample quantities in water).

Our drinking water treatment unit **"GOOD WATER"** is reliable and safe, it effectively restores the natural properties of water.

The **main** advantages for you are:

- healthy, clean, soft water from your own tap
- minimum cost of drinking water - under 5 cents per liter
- full automatic, reliable and controllable operational mode
- the highest quality due to the use of the best materials.

99 % of harmful substances, such as

- aluminum, antibiotics, arsenic, asbestos,
- benzene, chlorine, DDT, fluorides herbicides, hormones,
- lime, copper, medications, nitrates, PAH (polycyclic aromatic hydrocarbons, which, based on information from reliable sources, cause cancer), pentachlorophenol, pesticides, fungi, mercury, strontium,
- toluene, uranium, viruses and xylene

are eliminated from your water!

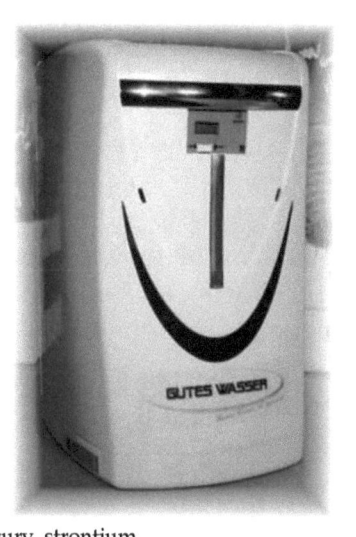

Price – 995 euros (installation not included)

LLC «GOOD WATER» (GUTES WASSER GMBH): AM BERGHOF, 5, 88630 PFULLENDORF
E-MAIL: KONTAKT@GUTESWASSER.INFO WEBSITE: WWW.GUTES-WASSER.INFO
TEL. 07552-933 79-0, FAX 07552-933 79 79

Chapter 7 - Strengthening Your Immune System

Do We Need Dietary Supplements Nowadays?

And What Do We Need to Know about Dietary Supplements?

Dietary supplements are food products which:

- are intended to supplement daily food,
- represent a concentrate of nutritional or other substances with a specific, for example, physiological effect (vitamins, minerals, including trace elements, amino acids, ferments, secondary plant substances, food fibres, plants or herbal extracts), taken either separately or in combination with other substances, and
- are packed in and marketed, amongst such forms as capsules, tablets, powder sachets and other forms, to be taken in pre-dispensed, limited doses.

Dietary supplements must have certain nutritional values. In the European Union, they are the most regulated food products. Information on such supplements must be submitted to the respective national authorities to test and approve them.

Isn't Regular Food Good Enough Anymore?

Experts of the Federal Institute for Risk Assessment (BfR) say that healthy people who consume balanced diet food do not need any dietary supplements. Balanced diet food intake guarantees that the human body gets all the necessary nutrients. That is why there's no need for additional dietary supplements.

Chapter 7 - Strengthening Your Immune System

On the other hand, a deficient, unbalanced diet cannot be fixed with the help of dietary supplements[13]. Only in some cases, rather infrequent ones in Germany, can targeted enrichment of daily rations with certain nutrients appear to be justified.

The latter statement by the Institute's experts requires clarification. f you read my further considerations, both you and I will surely question the information we are fed, namely, whether it is unbiased and trustworthy. Or does the referred institution establish to protect consumers' rights and health, or withhold the truth as was the case with drinking water (see page 162), so as to avoid causing fear and insecurity among the population?

People do not obviously benefit from that.

Without allowing anyone to deceive us, let's face the reality, face the truth.

Why Doesn't Our Body Get All the Necessary Nutrients, Though We Are Made to Believe Otherwise?

The main reason is mineral depletion of soil

For many years now, there have been a number of reports compiled on the lack of important nutrients, first and foremost, minerals and trace elements, in our daily food. As soil is both intensively cultivated and affected by acid rains, it does not receive minerals like zinc, iodine, chromium, selenium, magnesium, molybdenum, germanium, manganese, as well as some other vital substances. It is impossible to grow healthy plants which are rich in nutrients on such soils that have been depleted of minerals.

---

13) Source: Federal Institute for Risk Assessment (Bundesinstitut für Risikobewertung, BfR), Thielallee 88-92, 14195 Berlin, http://bfr.bund.de

Chapter 7 - Strengthening Your Immune System

So a human being does not get the necessary vitamins from vegetables and fruits.

Prof. Dr. med. Heinz Liesen, a nutrition expert, gives another reason for the lack of nutrients in plants: "The growth of plants is so much hastened by cultivation and genetic alterations that they cannot, or have no time, to develop important nutrients (Welt am Sonntag newspaper, 08.31.1997). Quality is sacrificed for quantity.

Other impacts, for instance, through acid rains, chemical fertilizers and pesticides lead to severe soil demineralization. This results in significantly lower soil natural fertility, which is determined by the presence of organic substances and minerals. Today, it is almost impossible to imagine agricultural activities free of chemicals. Research carried out by the UN in 1992 showed a sharp decrease in mineral substances contained in the soil on all continents over the last 100 years[14].

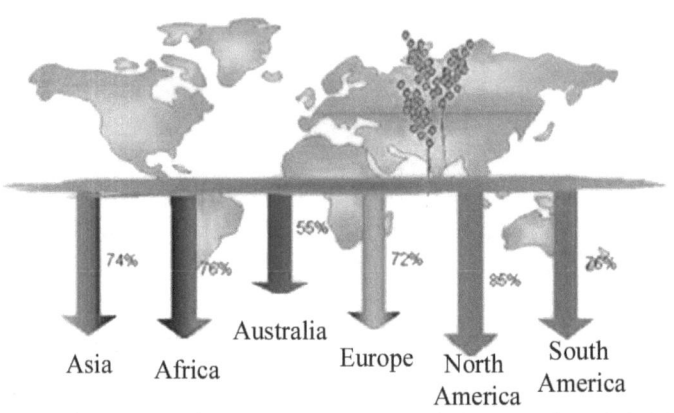

Region	Depletion
Asia	74%
Africa	76%
Australia	55%
Europe	72%
North America	85%
South America	76%

Source: the UN Earth Summit report, Rio de Janeiro, Brazil, 1992.

Soil mineral depletion over the last 100 years

14) Dr.med.John Switzer's website www.ein-langes-leben.de, Ayurveda Health and Beauty Centre in the Hotel Residence Starnberger See, Feldafing Germany.

Chapter 7 - Strengthening Your Immune System

Separate research conducted by the Ciba-Geigy Company for 11 years showed a clear reduction in various vitally important nutrients in vegetables and fruits. Most plants have seen the level of their mineral substances reduced by 40% on average.

Plants like spinach and broccoli find to have even greater reduction. Namely, spinach saw magnesium reduced by 68%, while broccoli had calcium reduced by 68% (Welt am Sonntag newspaper, 08.31.1997). Between 1986 and 1996 the amount of zinc provided by food that cultivated in Germany was reduced by 20%-25% (Source: Trace Elements and Electrolytes Journal, Vol. 15, No. 2, 1998).

Independent research work carried out in the USA, Canada, Great Britain and many other countries shows that the content of nutrients in our daily food has been significantly reduced in recent decades. The tables given below demonstrate a reduction in the content of nutrients based on the example of broccoli and potato sold in Canada from 1951 to 1999.

Broccoli	Calcium (mg)	Iron (mg)	Vitamin A (IU)	Vitamin C (mg)
1951	130,00	1,30	3500	104,0
1972	87,78	0,78	2500	90,0
1999	48,30	0,86	1542	93,5
Change (%)	-62,85	-33,85	-55,94	-10,10

Chapter 7 - Strengthening Your Immune System

Potato	Calcium (mg)	Iron (mg)	Vitamin A (IU)	Vitamin C (mg)
1951	11,00	0,70	20,00	17,00
1972	5,74	0,49	0,00	16,39
1999	7,97	0,30	0,00	7,25
Changes in %	-27,55	-57,14	-100	-57,35

The fact that a number of trace elements, such as zinc, selenium and iodine, cannot actually be found in soil, has been well-known to scientists for years[15].

Research by the German Nutrition Society (Deutsche Gesellschaft fur Ernahrung, DGE) shows that the magnesium level in daily food is approximately 18% lower than it should be according to actual nutritional value tables. Thus, today we suffer from a lack of magnesium. Besides, severe deficiencies in an additional 60 minerals and trace elements present in the human blood are of great importance.

In Germany people obtain, on average, just 35 mcg of selenium from food. However, many dietitians say that the selenium intake for a human should be 200 mcg. Selenium protects cells from oxidation by free radicals, from cancer, environmental toxins and heavy metals.

Recent studies done in the USA ("Cancer Prevention Diet") showed that daily intake of selenium in small doses can reduce the chances of cancer by 50%.

---
15) Further information on this problem can be found in:
- Vegetables Without Vitamins. Life Extension Magazine, March 2001. http://www.lef.org.magazine/mag2001/mar2001_report_vegetables.html
- Changes in USDA Food Composition Data for 43 Garden Crops, 1950 to 1999. Donald R. Davis, PhD, FACN, Melvin D. Epp, PhD and Hugh D. Riordan, MD. Journal of the American College of Nutrition, Vol. 23, No. 6, 669-682 (2004). http://www.jacn.org/cgi/content/abstract/23/6/669

Chapter 7 - Strengthening Your Immune System

Unfortunately, this data is totally ignored, as it does not fit into the framework of the pharmaceutical industry and conventional medicine. And billions are still spent on studies in chemotherapy and genetic engineering.

Unlike chemicals and genes, mineral substances such as selenium cannot be patented. <u>That is why no one is interested in them.</u>

Other Reasons for Lack of Vital Nutrients In Common Foods

Today, common foods have become junk foods, nothing but energy sources deprived of important substances. Namely, chemical compounds and elements which are vitally important for the body and cannot be independently synthesized by it from food and other sources like water, fats or amino acids.

Eating Less Does Not Mean Requiring Fewer Nutrients

About 50 years ago people were much more involved in physical work, moving around, and so they could, and had to, eat more. Due to this, they also obtained more vitamins and vitally important substances.

Nowadays a human does not need – and actually should not! – eat that much, as the body does not require so much energy, <u>but it needs as many vitamins as back then.</u> As a matter of fact, this is one of the reasons why older people, who do not eat much, often lack vitamins and mineral **nutrients**.

Ready-Made Food

Ready-made foods should be avoided, as the devil avoids holy water!, regardless of the manufacturer and place of sale.

Chapter 7 - Strengthening Your Immune System

More often than not, eating in canteens and cafes is nothing but "stuffing oneself". Ready-made food has nothing in common with food products!

Microwave Oven

A microwave oven that seems a practical kitchen appliance at first sight, is a real "killer for vitamins and vitally important substances". It takes only a couple of minutes to successfully destroy those few substances necessary for our body, which our dishes still contain.

Apparently, you now know our opinion on microwave ovens and what we did with it.

Stress Factors

The stress factors of modern life have considerably increased, mainly due to our inadequate, unnatural lifestyle which **additionally** increases the body's need for vitally important substances.

Today We Are Hungry Despite Being "Chock-Full"

While in the past, people suffered from a real lack of nutrition, today we are hungry, figuratively speaking, despite being "chock-full", experiencing overabundance, because we pay too much attention to quantity, external appearance, taste and price, paying too little attention to quality and the internal content of our food products!

Conclusions to Be Drawn Personally

What conclusions can be drawn from all above? Well, our daily food should include fresh fruits and vegetables as much

Chapter 7 - Strengthening Your Immune System

as possible! And more attention should be paid to quality, not price!

When taking dietary supplements, it is crucial that they are of high biological quality and contain ingredients which meet the requirements of nutritional science, in order to be fully accepted by the body. Nothing else matters.

With regard to vitamins, focus on their major difference - so-called "biological effectiveness", that is, whether the vitamins are produced chemically or obtained naturally and/or biologically.

> *Talk to your naturopath or doctor educated in naturopathy, about issues related to taking dietary supplements, especially those applied in big doses, or eating food items that contain supplements. In any case, ask them if they are well up on these issues. Otherwise, your doctor may appear to know about nutrition as much – or as little – as you do.*

Chapter 7 - Strengthening Your Immune System

Remedy Detox-Pulver

Clinoptilolite-Zeolite Is a Volcanic Material

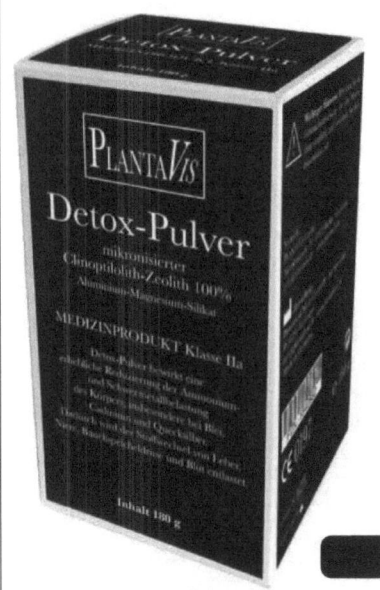

For your health and detoxification.

✓ Eases the burden on the metabolism in the liver, kidneys, pancreas and blood.

✓ Detox-Pulver Remedy by Planta Vis reduces internal contamination with ammonium and heavy metals, particularly with lead, cadmium and mercury.

IIa Class Remedy

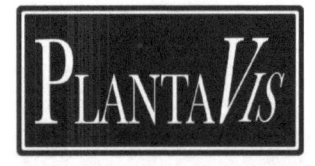

19 Rosa-Luxemburg Str.
14482 Potsdam,
Germany
www.plantavis.de

PLANTA*Vis*

www.plantavis.de

CHAPTER 8

The Special Juice

⌘

Treatment Cornerstones

> *Important preliminary remark: vegetable juice is, along with herbal teas, the most important component, virtually the foundation, of cancer treatment. It is not for nothing that Breuss also calls the treatment the "juice treatment".*

In this Chapter I would like to tell you more about this juice.

Shall I Press Juice Myself or Buy Ready-made Juice?

Breuss vegetable juice can be bought ready-made, or you can press it at home by yourself.

- Who should press the juice at home?
- When should the juice be pressed at home?
- Who should buy ready-made juice?
- When should the ready-made juice be bought?
- What does Rudolf Breuss say about this?
- What is the author's opinion on this?

What Are the Benefits of Juice Pressed at Home

- Let us at first give the floor to Rudolf Breuss who says that in case of severe cancers it is necessary, if possible,

Chapter 8 - The Special Juice

to press the juice daily from organically grown vegetables. And now let me ask, "Do you have a minor cancer?"

• When pressing by yourself (under "pressing by yourself" I mean that the patient, he or she, presses the juice), the patient can be newly motivated each day – and make his or her quality by himself or herself.

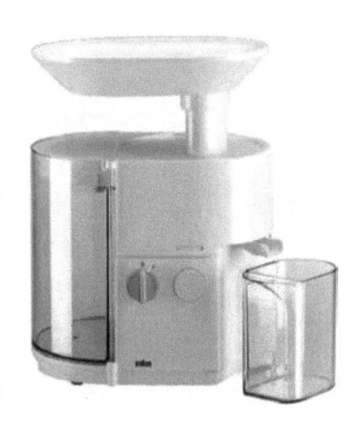

• Those patients who make the juice at home can spare save a few Euros during the treatment, since vegetables for the juice are cheaper than a ready-made product. But in this case you should not take the work into account!

• Only those who press the juice by themselves can easily benefit from the solution that I suggest below if you don't like vegetable juice (anymore) or if you cannot stand raw potato.

• The fact that the shelf life of ready-made juice on offer is two years makes me wary, so I tend to press juice myself.

What Are the Benefits of Ready-made Juice

• Those who use ready-made juice, certainly save time needed for its preparation which is particularly crucial if the patient has to keep up with his full workload during the treatment.

• If no fresh organically grown vegetables are available (beetroot, carrot, celery, radish and potato), which is often the case when they are out of season, then in my view the only solution can be ready-made juice. During my struggle

Chapter 8 - The Special Juice

against cancer, however (in April and May, i.e. out of harvesting season), I always pressed the juice myself, even if the products were not organically grown. And I would also recommend you do the same.

- Upon my inquiry, Biotta-AG told me that it does not intend to be associated with cancer by producing the "the Breuss vegetable juice mix" developed according to Rudolf Breuss's original recipe. So, press it yourselves!

How You Should Drink the Juice

Rudolf Breuss writes, "The patient may go up to one half liter but this is not necessary". As to the quantity of the vegetable juice, "The less juice the patient drinks the better".

I drank one half liter in two portions: one quarter of a liter in small sips in the first half of the day and another quarter liter in the second half of the day, also in small sips. This split was good for me – during the treatment I felt quite vigorous.

> *Tip 1: if you feel undernourished or weak and low in spirits during the treatment, it is better to drink this one half liter. Provided that you can tolerate this juice and feel it agrees well with you.*

> *Tip 2: if you don't feel better, you may want to stop taking the juice for one day, so as to let your palate and taste buds recover.*

Important: always mix the juice with saliva. In this case, if you slowly sip this small quantity (of juice and teas), it gets broken down, thereby helping your digestive tract.

Chapter 8 - The Special Juice

Making Your Own Vegetable Juice

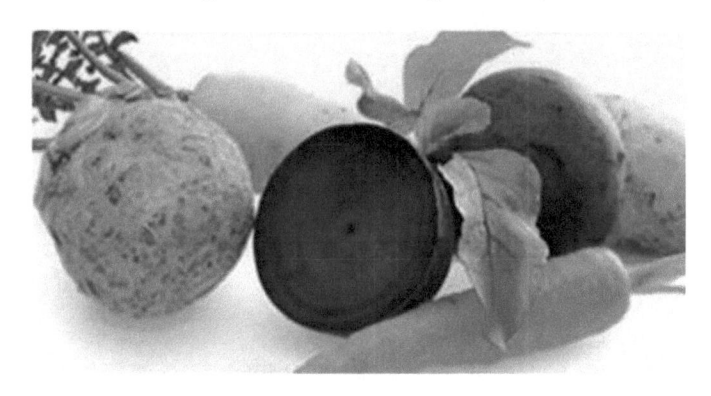

Beet root, carrot, celeriac, radish and potato

The daily juice mix during cancer treatment consists of five ingredients:

- 300 g beetroot
- 100 g carrots
- 100 g celery root
- 30 g radish
- 1 potato, the size of an egg.

From these vegetables you can press about ½ a liter of juice (depending on the season and the juice extractor). It is vital to drink only 1/8 to ¼ liter of juice per day. **If this amount of vegetables does not produce enough juice (which is entirely possible due to seasonal conditions), you need to increase it.**

Chapter 8 - The Special Juice

Proceed as follows: clean the vegetables but do not peel them. If the potato is too old because of the season, you can remove the coarsest knobs; cut the vegetables into thin sticks so that they fit into the feeding chute of the extractor, press them with the extractor and then filter the juice through a linen cloth as for each quarter liter of juice there is always, according to experience, a tablespoon of sediment.

This sediment would <u>serve as food for cancer!</u>

If you wish to use a tea strainer instead of a linen cloth, test its suitability this way: filter the freshly pressed vegetable juice through the strainer and then through a linen cloth. If there is no sediment in the cloth, the strainer is suitable. Otherwise, unfortunately, it is not.

The same applies to modern super juicers with nano-filters or similar filters. Always do the **linen cloth test!**

You must know how the juice ingredients are effective:

- Beetroot is helpful in fighting cancer
- Carrot contains carotene, which is essential for the human body,
- Celeriac contains phosphorus, which is essential for the human body,
- Radish and potato juices are vital for the liver.

Important: press juice every day and drink it at room temperature. It should not be put in the refrigerator!

In the container, usually a glass in which the juice flows from the extractor, there is always some sediment that must be left

Chapter 8 - The Special Juice

there. As a rule, it is potato starch, which is the reason why some patients don't like the juice. So take my **tip: do not stir the juice!**

On the Subject of Potato

"It is not compulsory to add potato juice to the juice mixture", says Rudolf Breuss. Not everyone tolerates potato or likes its taste in the vegetable juice mixture. So it is reassuring to know that Breuss offers a substitute: potatoes' skin tea.
I have always added potato to my juice. Despite this fact, I generally enjoyed the juice.

"Instead of adding potato to the juice mixture", says Breuss in the same context, "you can drink a cup of potatoes' skin tea each day. This tea is to be slowly sipped cold". Prepare this tea in the following way: boil a handful of raw potato skins in two cups of water for 2-4 minutes. Then sieve the tea.

However, in case of <u>liver cancer</u> potato juice is **absolutely essential**! If you do not tolerate raw potato then in this case, also slowly sip one cup of cold potatoes' skin tea per day. If the potatoes' skin tea does not taste good ("good" is in this respect, in the true sense of the word, a matter of personal taste), then your liver does not need it, so you do not have to drink it.

If You Don't Like Vegetable Juice (Anymore)

I have noticed that many patients find vegetable juice delicious; however, some do not like it at all. In some cases, this can be so bad as to cause vomiting. Breuss also knew this, but, unfortunately his book contains no specific reference to possible solutions.

Chapter 8 - The Special Juice

I heard a story from a grandson of Breuss as to what once happened to his grandfather: *old Breuss wanted to demonstrate his juice treatment to a married couple who visited him in his house (Breuss' book "Cancer/ leukemia" had not yet been written). For this purpose, he prepared freshly-pressed vegetable juice. The guests tasted a sip, and the woman threw up the juice. Thereupon Breuss sliced an orange in half, squeezed out the juice, poured it through a linen cloth and added it to the vegetable juice. Both patients tasted it. Not only did nausea disappear, but they also liked the juice.*

Based on this story and other considerations and tests, I developed vegetable juices to everyone's taste. They all contain the ingredients permitted by Breuss:

Vegetable Juice with Orange

A favourite of Breuss. It tastes (for me) extremely good and is easy to prepare. Press vegetable juice following the general instructions above. But before filtering the juice through a linen cloth, toss half or a whole orange (depending on the ripeness of the orange and season of the year, the volume of the juice can vary) into the feeding chute. Then filter the pulp and enjoy a delicious drink: vegetable juice with orange.

If you drink ready-made juice, add to it the appropriate amount of freshly pressed and filtered (through a linen cloth) orange juice and stir. *Your vegetable juice with orange is ready.*

Vegetable Juice with Sauerkraut

Some people like it, but I don't. However, it is worth trying: press vegetable juice following the general instructions above and add per glass at least one teaspoon of biological sauerkraut juice which you already use to help digestion (see "Bowel

Chapter 8 - The Special Juice

Cleansing", Chapter 6). Cheers!

If you drink ready-made juice, add to it the appropriate amount of biological sauerkraut juice and stir. *Your vegetable juice with sauerkraut is also ready.*

Vegetable Juice with Lemon

Vegetable juice with lemon tastes especially good for many patients. My recommendations for preparation are as follows: press vegetable juice following the general instructions above and then add to it the juice of half or a whole lemon (depending on the ripeness of the lemon and season of the year, the volume of the juice can vary). Thereafter, just as always, filter the mixture through a linen cloth, and vegetable juice with lemon is ready! If you drink ready-made juice, add to it the appropriate amount of freshly pressed and filtered through a linen cloth the lemon juice and stir. *Your vegetable juice with lemon is also ready.*

Chapter 8 - The Special Juice

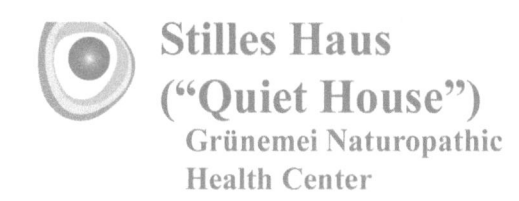

Stilles Haus ("Quiet House")
Grünemei Naturopathic Health Center

Management
Dr. Christian T. Grünemei is a homeopathic practitioner and social educationalist. Dr. Grünemei's 12-year experience of supporting and treating guests and patients guarantee his effectiveness and professionalism.

Main Directions and Practices
Holistic diagnosis, consultations, nutritional therapy, fasting, intestinal cleanse and detoxification, naturopathy. Movement therapy, meditation.
We also offer the Breuss fasting therapy based on an individual approach.
Medically supervised programs are available on request.

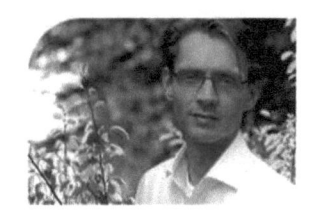

The House
We offer our guests spacious, light-filled rooms with a private sun terrace. At your service is an extensive range of equipment, sauna, massage rooms, a library and the Internet. The Center is located in the wonderful Kellerwald-Edersee National Park; the surroundings contain a whole network of walking trails.
The "Quiet House" Naturopathic Health Center is certified in accordance with the EU Eco-Regulation for catering.

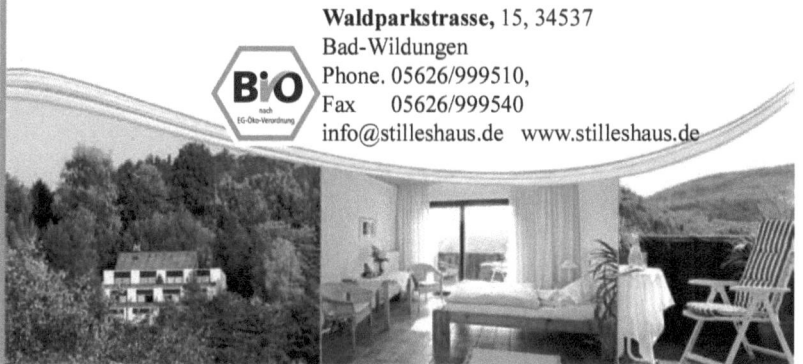

Waldparkstrasse, 15, 34537 Bad-Wildungen
Phone. 05626/999510,
Fax   05626/999540
info@stilleshaus.de   www.stilleshaus.de

CHAPTER 9

SPECIAL BROTHS AND TINCTURES

⌘

Important Components of Effective Treatment

> *Important preliminary remark: broths and tinctures, alongside vegetable juices and teas, are important components of cancer treatment.*

In this Chapter, I would like to familiarize you with preparation of these *broths*, onion broth, and for those who cannot tolerate this soup or have liver or gall-bladder complaints, broth of bean pods. This Chapter will also take a look at hawthorn tincture.

Onion Broth

During the therapy, one may, or even should, eat one or two bowls of onion broth a day (in the afternoon, <u>not in the evening</u>). Take only the liquid, not the onion! If you do not like this broth, you can skip it or just have one bowl at noon.

Note: before you decide to skip this broth untested, taste it! For many, including myself, onion broth has been and is a culinary highlight of the day!!!

Preparation: cut an onion the size of a lemon into small pieces together with the brown outer skin and fry it in a little (!) vegetable fat or oil untill it is golden brown. My wife added

Chapter 9 - Special Broths and Tinctures

some drops of olive oil to the onion broth – but only a few drops! Then add some ½ a liter of cold water and simmer until the onion is well-cooked – i.e. around 20 minutes. Finally, add a vegetable bouillon cube or vegetable broth[16] and stir well. Pass the broth through a sieve[17] and drink only the clear liquid – without the onion!

Important: with liver or gall bladder cancer never eat a whole bowl of onion broth in one sitting! It is best to drink or "eat" around 10 tablespoons of warm broth every hour.

> *Tip: do not throw away the onions: they may be eaten (of course, not by the patient undergoing the treatment!) as onion soup; not only are they delicious but also helpful, according to Rudolf Breuss, e.g. against bone decalcification (osteoporosis).*

Broth of Bean Pods

(Note: it is only an alternative in very particular cases)

If you have problems with your **liver or gall-bladder** and cannot stand onion soup, you should cook broth of bean pods instead of onion soup.

During the therapy, one may, or even should, consume one or

---

16) I am often asked which broths (those that come in either pouches or cubes) are the right ones. My answer is: it should definitely be a vegetable broth or vegetable bouillon.
Search the stores for organic products and try various tastes on offer. For it is going to be your culinary highlight of the day!
And as broth is mainly responsible for the taste of onion soup, the proof of the broth is in the eating – and it's common knowledge that tastes differ. You have six weeks time!
17) Passing through a sieve is understood as pouring liquid from one container to another through a sieve. This will prevent tea leaves, etc. from getting into the cup.

Chapter 9 - Special Broths and Tinctures

two bowls of broth of bean pods a day.
 Note: take only the liquid, not the bean pods! If you do not like this broth, you can skip it or just have one bowl at noon.

Preparation: cut dried bean pods (from your own vegetable garden?) into small pieces and fry one heaped tablespoon of them until golden brown in a little vegetable fat or oil. Then add ½ a liter of cold water and simmer until the bean pods are well-cooked. Finally, add a vegetable bouillon cube and stir well once again. Pass the broth through a sieve and drink only the clear liquid!

> *Tip:* if bean pods are not available (according to my observation, it is a common problem when beans are out of season), you can prepare the broth with commercially available ground bean pods. Put one heaped tablespoon of ground bean pods into a pot, add around ½ a liter of cold water and simmer for 20 minutes. Finally, add one teaspoon of clear broth or a vegetable bouillon cube and stir well. Then pass through a sieve and drink only the clear liquid.

Hawthorn Tincture

To support the functioning of the work, take 20 to 40 hawthorn drops <u>in the morning</u> (depending on the patient's body size and weight).

> I am regularly asked whether the alcohol contained in hawthorn drops is not harmful. This is not the case. The daily intake is so low that no undesirable side effects would be expected.

CHAPTER 10

Special Teas

⌘

Another Treatment Cornerstone

> *Important preliminary remark: teas, along with the vegetable juice, are the* most important elements *of the treatment and, therefore, are not a matter of free choice. The intake of teas recommended for various cancer types is* mandatory.

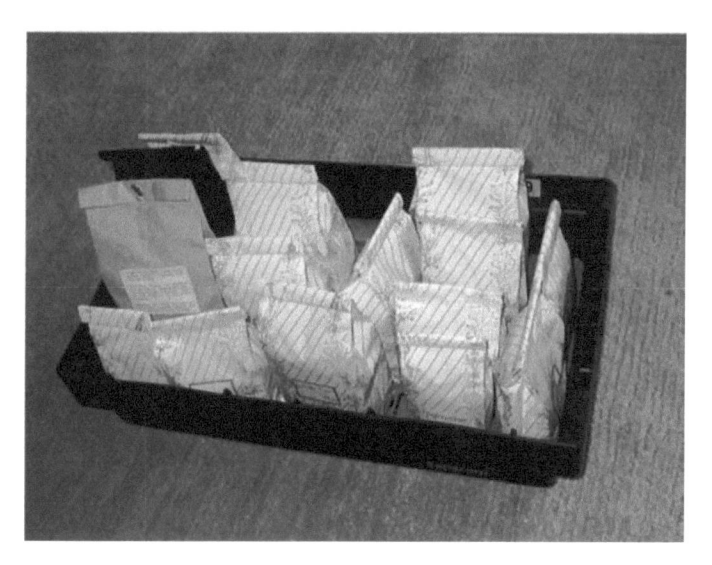

Your tea supply for the treatment looks something like this
All teas must be taken <u>without sugar</u> and also <u>without milk</u>!

Chapter 10 - Special Teas

They are prepared with still mineral water or with regular tap water, the way you usually make tea.

All teas should be taken in sips and mixed with saliva.

An exception is made for the "Breuss original sage tea" in the Breuss mixture and the special tea mix which one can – and even should - drink when thirsty. And the more, the better!

Breuss' book does not give any details about the size of a cup. Often he even omits the cup as a unit of size and speaks simply about hot water.
I am 187 cm tall and my weight is 105 kg; thus, I used large cups (250 ml). For most patients, a normal cup (150 ml) would be sufficient.

When speaking about teas we often mention a "pinch": it is the amount you can hold between your thumb and two fingers, for a coarsely-chopped herb. For a finely-chopped herb, take half a rounded tablespoon.

In the appendix you will find labels for the most frequently used teas which you can cut out or, perhaps better, copy and stick on the respective tea containers. Thus, you will not have to take this book each time when you prepare your teas.

When is it better to prepare teas? Depending on the time available you can do it on evenings (if you have to leave early in the morning), or mornings (if you have time for this), or, depending on the kind of tea, partly evenings, partly mornings. The only condition is that kidney tea, which you will drink in the first three weeks, should be taken on mornings right after hawthorn drops and sipped cold. Therefore, you will need enough time for this tea to cool.

I prepared all teas in the morning. With the result that half a cup of kidney tea I drank right after getting up was 24 hours old. On the other hand, all other teas were absolutely fresh. And these warm teas (for example, marigold tea) seemed amazingly tasty to me.

Infusions (Brews, Teas) to Be Taken for <u>All</u> Cancer Types

Kidney Tea
- Tea necessary for <u>all</u> cancer types –

Mix this tea yourself, using:

- 30 g horsetail (botanical name: Equisetum arvense),
- 20 g stinging nettle (botanical name: Urtica dioica, it is best collected by yourself in springtime!),
- 15 g knotgrass (botanical name: Polygonum aviculare), and
- 10 g St. John's wort (botanical name: Hypericum perforatum).

Using the ratio above, you should mix this so-called kidney tea in advance and keep it in store, mix it yourself so that you will know what it contains! This quantity is sufficient for one person for approximately three weeks, since kidney tea is to be taken for <u>only the first three weeks</u>

Preparation: for three half cups of kidney tea, take a pinch of tea (the amount you can hold between your thumb and two fingers), put it in a pot, pour one cup of boiling water and steep for 10 minutes. Then strain out the tea leaves and set aside the liquid. Add another two cups of hot water to the tea leaves, and boil them for 10 minutes: after this, strain the tea and blend the two liquids.

Why is this tea prepared like this? Kidney tea contains 5 substances which can not be boiled as they are destroyed through cooking. It also contains a sixth substance (silicic acid), which can be extracted only by boiling tea leaves for another 10 minutes.

> *Tip: due to the fact that this tea is very healthy, Breuss advises to take this three-week treatment three or four times a year, however, with intervals of at least two weeks.*

Marigold Tea
- Tea necessary **for all cancer types** -

For a change, it is recommended to take **marigold tea** (botanical name: Calendula officinalis) which according to Breuss has been known as an anti-cancer medication since time immemorial. One to two teaspoons (2-3 g) are poured with hot water (some 150 ml) and after steep for 10 minutes strained through a tea strainer.

This tea, in combination with sage tea and cranesbill tea – or herb Robert tea - (but please do not mix them!) stimulates the activity of excretory organs by suppressing the so-called viromycose, disturbances of the cellular respiration processes in the blood (Breuss' original book, page 49).

Sage Tea
- Tea necessary **for all cancer types** -

This tea, the "Breuss original sage tea", consists of several ingredients:

Chapter 10 - Special Teas

- Tea from sage leaves, and
- Mixture of additional herbal teas.

To make preparation easier, make the tea in advance, mixing the ingredients below in the proportion 1:1:1, that is

- 100 g St. John's wort (botanical name: Hypericum perforatum),
- 100 g peppermint (botanical name: Mentha piperita)
- 100 g lemon balm (botanical name: Melissa officinalis)

I have called this mixture "tea mix – sage tea ingredients", see "Tea Labels", Appendix 5. Due to its significant volume, you can certainly start with mixing, for example, just 50 grams of each herb.

Preparation: put three, at the most four teaspoons of sage (better less than more, otherwise it will be too strong) in one liter of boiling water and **boil for exactly three minutes**. Once the sage tea has been boiled for three minutes, turn off the heat source and add 3-4 pinches of the "tea mix – sage tea ingredients". Then let everything steep for another 10 minutes.

Each day, I prepared not 1 liter, but 1. 5 liters of sage tea. You may drink this tea as much as you want, the more the better. This tea in combination with marigold and cranesbill teas – or herb Robert tea - (but please do not mix them!) stimulates the activity of excretory organs, having a positive impact on toxin elimination and anti-inflammatory effects.

Chapter 10 - Special Teas

Breuss considers sage tea the most important of all herbal teas! You should drink it throughout your life.

> *Background information: sage contains a large amount of essential oils, which are very useful for gargling, but these oils can not be ingested. So it is necessary to boil sage tea for exactly three minutes.*
> *After three minutes the oils are boiled away, thus releasing the enzymes which are **vital** for the health of all glands, bone marrow and intervertebral discs.*

For gargling (that has nothing to do with cancer treatment) 1. 5 teaspoon of sage leaves (botanical name: Salvia officinalis) should be steeped for 10 minutes in 150 ml of hot water.

> *Important: on most tea packets there is, unfortunately, no indication of how to make sage tea in the correct way. This applies not only to the special preparation of the Rudolf Breuss sage tea (taken with the "tea mix – sage tea ingredients"), but also to regular preparation of tea from sage leaves only!*
> *Therefore, it is always important to boil sage tea for three minutes and not simply steep it for 10 minutes, the way it is generally indicated on packages/bags.*

Cranesbill (Herb Robert) Tea
- Tea necessary **for all cancer types** –

Steep a pinch of leaves of cranesbill (herb Robert, Geranium Robertianum) in a cup of hot water for 10 minutes. Slowly sip one cup of cold tea each day (over the course of the day).

Cranesbill tea is vital for all types of cancer, especially if you

Chapter 10 - Special Teas

have received radiation treatment, because the tea contains a small amount of radium. This tea, in combination with sage and marigold teas, stimulates the activity of excretory organs by helping one's kidneys to eliminate toxins.

Special Tea Mix
(A term I invented myself)
- Tea necessary **for all cancer types** –

This special tea mix is recommended for prevention of lime and calcium deficiency in case of bone and lung cancer; however, it is also useful in fighting all other cancer types.

For treatment purposes, make the tea in advance, mixing equal parts of the ingredients below:

- 100 g ribwort plantain or broadleaf plantain (botanical name: Plantago lanceolata or Plantago major),
- 100 g Iceland moss (botanical name: Cetraria islandica),
- 100 g lungwort (botanical name: Pulmonaria officinalis)
- 100 g ground ivy (botanical name: Glechoma hederacea),
- 100 g mullein (botanical name: Verbascum densiflorum)
- 100 g Ligusticum mutellina (botanical name: Meum mutellina) – see Chapter 11 "Cancer Treatment Shopping List".

Due to its significant volume, you can certainly start with mixing, for example, 50 grams of each herb.

Chapter 10 - Special Teas

Breuss says that not all these six herbs have to be included in this mix. Taking this into account, it will not jeopardize successful therapy if you can not find Ligusticum mutellina.

Preparation: take one good pinch of Special Tea Mix per cup of hot water (approx. 150 ml), put it in hot water and steep for 10 minutes. Prepare and drink at least one liter of this tea each day (this corresponds to about 6-7 pinches).

You can drink as much of this tea as you want, the more the better. Thus, prepare a sufficiently large amount of it

> *Tip: it is not improbable that during treatment you will face situations when everyone is drinking in company. However, since water (as well as all other drinks) is forbidden, I used to take a thermos bottle with the previously brewed herbal tea and ask the host or a waiter to serve it to me as a "wine spritzer" (cold tea looks very similar to it).*

Additional Teas for <u>Specific</u> Cancer Types

Eyebright Tea
- To use solely in case of **eye cancer** -

Steep a pinch of eyebright (botanical name: Euphrasia rostkoviana) in a cup of hot water for 10 minutes. Drink this cup of cold eyebright tea per day, swallowed slowly, in addition to the teas above, which are taken for all cancer types.

Valerian Tea
- To use solely in case of **stomach cancer**
and <u>additional nervous stomach</u> –

If a patient with gastric cancer has an irritable bowel syndrome, apart from wormwood tea (botanical name: Artemisia absinthium) or centaurium tea (Latin: Centaurium erythraea), see chapters focusing on these teas, he should also take one cup of valerian tea with wormwood a day.

Wormwood here is taken to mean the medicinal plant of Artemisa absinthium, and not an alcoholic beverage (though in German both words sound identical – *Wermut*).

Preparation: place ½ a teaspoon of valerian root in a cup of water and boil for 3 minutes, then take a strainer, put into it a pinch of wormwood and for three seconds pour the tea through the strainer into another cup.

Chapter 10 - Special Teas

Pimpernel Tea
*- To use solely in case of **cancer of gums, lips, tongue, neck lymph nodes and larynx** -*

In case of cancer of gums, lips, tongue, neck lymph nodes and larynx, rinse your mouth and throat with pimpernel tea (Latin: Pimpinella). Boil a teaspoon of pimpernel tea in a cup of water for three minutes several times a day.

Gargle your mouth and throat with a tablespoon of pimpernel tea and then spit it out. Do the same with the second tablespoonful of the tea. After gargling your mouth and throat with the third tablespoonful, swallow the tea. Do this several times a day.

Potatoes' Skin Tea
*- To use solely in case of **liver cancer** -*

Patients with liver cancer should additionally drink two warm or cold cups of potatoes' skin tea per day, taking small and slow sips.
Put a handful of raw potato skins in two cups of hot water and boil for 2-4 minutes. If this tea tastes agreeable, then it will be good for your liver. If it tastes disagreeable, then you would better not drink it.

Lemon Balm Tea
*- To use solely in case of **cerebral tumor** -*

In case of cerebral tumor, also drink one or two cups of cold lemon balm tea per day, taking small and slow sips. It may be crimson (scarlet) bee balm (botanical name: Monarda didyma) or lemon balm (balm mint) (botanical name: Melissa officinalis), or their mixture. Steep one pinch of herb in hot water for 10 minutes.

Chapter 10 - Special Teas

Celandine Tea
- To use solely in case of **skin cancer** -

Put a pinch of greater celandine herb into one cup of hot water and steep for 10 minutes. Apply to the skin still lukewarm. If there is no fresh greater celandine juice (Chelidonium majus) available, for example, in winter, you can swab or cleanse the affected area with celandine tea or celandine tincture, but only around the affected area.

You can also order a living plant from herb traders and cultivate it over these 6 weeks. Fresh is just fresh!

Silver Lady's Mantle and Lady's Mantle Tea
- To use solely in case of **breast, ovarian and uterine cancers**-

Take one cup of cold tea made from silvery lady's mantle (botanical name: Alchemilla alpina) or lady's mantle (botanical name: Alchemilla vulgaris) with a pinch of yellow dead nettle (botanical name: Lamium galeobdolon) or white dead nettle, also known as blind nettle (botanical name: Lamium album) per day, swallowed slowly. To prepare, take a pinch of silvery lady's mantle tea or lady's mantle, or their mixture, add a small pinch of lamium and steep in a cup of hot water for 10 minutes.

> *Tip:* if possible, purchase all four of these herbs – silvery lady's mantle, lady's mantle, yellow and white dead nettle, and mix them in the proportion 1:1:0.5:0.5 in advance. For brewing, take a good pinch of this mixture for one cup.

Willow Herb Tea
- To use solely in case of **testicular and prostate cancer** –

Put a pinch of willow herb tea (Latin: Epilobii parvifloris concis) in each of two cups of hot water (one pinch for one cup) and steep for 10 minutes. Slowly sip these two cups of cold tea, in several sittings during the day.

Wormwood or Centaury Tea
- To use solely in case of **stomach cancer** -

In case of stomach cancer, you should additionally drink one cup of cold wormwood tea (botanical name: Artemisia absinthium) or centaury tea (botanical name: Centaurium erythraea) a day, taking small and slow sips.
Preparation: steep a small pinch of wormwood or centaury in a cup of hot water for only three seconds.

Wormwood Tea
- To use solely in case of **liver and gall bladder cancers** –

In case of liver and gall bladder cancers, take additionally one cup of warm or cold wormwood tea (botanical name: Artemisia absinthium) per day, taking small and slow sips.

Preparation: over the first five or six days, steep one small pinch of wormwood in a cup of hot water for 10 seconds. Starting from the seventh day, steep wormwood for only three seconds, otherwise the tea will be too strong!

Chapter 10 - Special Teas

Tea Preparation is a Matter of Organization

The production of both vegetable juices and herbal teas is actually not a complicated task. It may seem to be complicated at the beginning of the treatment. After several days it will become a familiar routine for you.

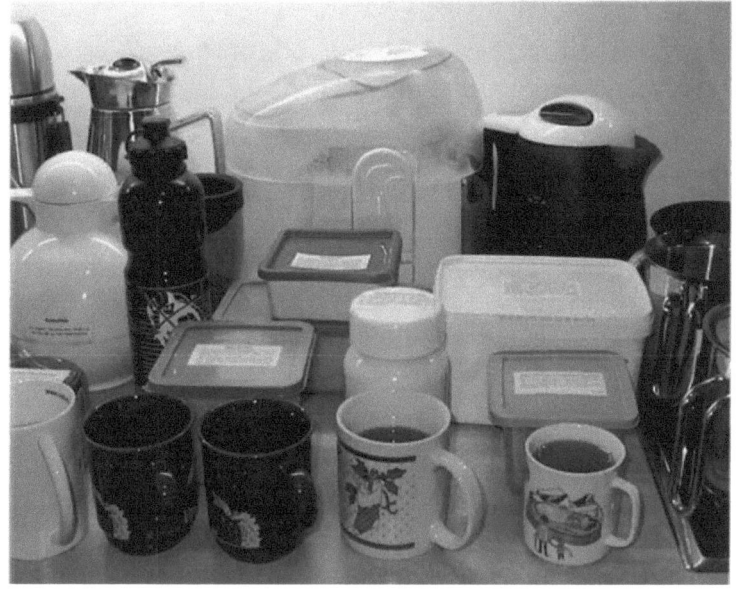

My "workspace" for making of herbal teas and vegetable juices

Below is the sequence of my tea-brewing activities:

- Boil a little more than one liter of water.

- During this time, put sage leaves into a pot and place the cups, as well as neatly labeled and sorted tea containers, behind them.

- Pour the boiling water on the sage leaves and allow them to simmering for three minutes.

- During this time boil another kettle of fresh water (my kettle holds 1. 7 l of water).

Chapter 10 - Special Teas

- In the meantime prepare thermos bottles and other containers (preheated so that the tea remains hot for a long time) and put into the cups which stand in front of "their" containers the prescribed quantity of herbal teas.

- The same applies to the pots with handles shown in the right: into the smaller one I put kidney tea and into the larger one – the special tea mix.

- In three minutes, I put the boiling sage tea aside, add the special sage mix and leave it to infuse for 10 minutes.

- By this time, the water in the kettle has reached boiling point, and I pour the water into the cups and the pot for kidney tea.

- Yet there is not enough boiling water to completely fill the pot with the special tea mix. Therefore, I put another kettle with fresh water on the hotplate in order to refill the mix.

- After sage tea has brewed for 10 minutes, I pour it into a ready-to-use small thermos bottle (0.5 liter). The remaining tea is poured into the tea cups – it will be taken hot.

- The remaining hot water is poured into the special tea mix.

- In the meantime, having brewed for 10 minutes, the kidney tea is strained and boiled for another 10 minutes.

- After the teas have brewed in the cups for 10 minutes, strain them using an additional large cup and place into the "storage area" opposite the described "workspace" in the kitchen, see photo below).

- After the special tea mix in the second pot with a handle has also brewed, I pour this tea - all of it or just a part - into a large thermos bottle, and the rest goes either into another thermos bottle, or into a bike water bottle shown on

Chapter 10 - Special Teas

the photo in the left, as a "wine spritzer" for a night out with friends. See Chapter 6, "Cancer Treatment on the Move".

The ready-to-drink kidney tea is poured into cups, and so the preparation of teas is complete. I repeatedly timed how long this entire process took me: 20 minutes.

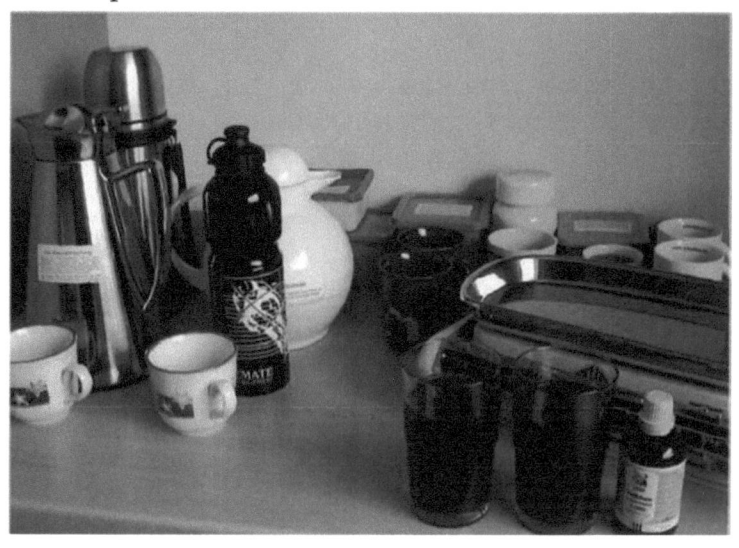

"Storage area" for ready-to-drink teas and vegetable juice

And now that we have come to talk about time: making of vegetable juice including cleaning the workspace (I did not wash utensils by hand – instead, I put them into the dishwasher) took me 15 minutes on average.

All in all, I spent a good half-hour on both processes - preparation of all herbal teas and making of fresh vegetable juice.

Chapter 10 - Special Teas

If the Teas No Longer Taste Good

At the beginning of the treatment herbal teas taste nice, especially when warm. Some of you will even find them delicious. But it can so happen that in the course of the treatment this will change. In this case you can try to diversify the treatment program. Experiment with your taste – you have an entire 42 days for that! However, you should use only the above-mentioned ingredients.

Tea with Lemon

Add to the cup of tea (whatever the type, it can be sage tea mix or special tea mix – try them out!) a few drops of a freshly-squeezed and strained lemon juice. It will change the taste of your tea considerably.

Teas with Various Strength

If tea is too strong, it can have a bitter taste and be not to everyone's liking. If tea is weakish, it tastes bland and flavorless. If having cooked and brewed tea exactly in accordance with my instructions, you do not like it (anymore), this may be due to the amount of tea used in relation to the volume of water. And this may in turn stem from the size of the cups used, "dimensions of fingers" of the pinch, or the condition of the tea leaves. These leaves can show considerable individual variations: one supplier can have them more powdered (crumbled), another – less powdered, with the result that the measure used may not comply with the instructions.

You may experiment with those teas that have an unpleasant taste by slightly changing the quantity of their ingredients, thereby making the tea weaker or stronger. It should be completely enjoyable and, of course, effective.

In any case, experimenting can be of great benefit. Don't forget that you have six weeks time for this.

CHAPTER 11

Cancer Treatment Shopping List

⌘

Arrangements First!

How Much Juice Vegetables Provide

In case your juicer does not extract enough juice out of the amount of vegetables (as some of them extract more juice than others), I suggest that you need to make the appropriate adjustments to the amount of vegetables you buy.

The same refers to the season, as undoubtedly, fresh vegetables yield more juice than those stored in a warehouse for a long time.

Posttreatment Use of Leftover Herbal Tea Leaves

If you have a small amount of any herbal tea left, it doesn't mean that you haven't taken enough of it – this leftover is a part of the plan.

To my mind, it is better to have some leftovers for posttreatment use, than to make additional orders and wait for days until they are delivered.

Even now from time to time I drink herbal teas that are leftovers from my treatment. Why not?

Chapter 11 - Cancer Treatment Shopping List

Treatment Shopping List
(just copy the list or cut it out and take it with you when out shopping)

Vegetables for juicing (greengrocer's, market place)	
Amount per week	Name
2,0 kg	Red beet (botanical name: Beta vulgaris)
1 bunch/pack/approx. 0.7 kg	Carrot (botanical name: Daucus carotta ssp. Sativus Apiaceae)
1 bulb approx. 0.7 kg	Celeriac (botanical name: Apium graveolens var. Rapaceum)
1 piece, at least 0.2 kg	Radish (botanical name: Raphanus sativus), red or white
1 net, or 7 egg-sized potatoes	Potato (botanical name: Solanum tuberosum subspecies tuberosum)

Breuss Vegetable Juice from Biotta I do not know of Biotta channels of distribution. That is why I'd like to draw your attention to my note on page 185. However, both companies indicated on page 220 will readily fulfill your order.	
Amount per course of treatment	Notes
21 liters (max. ½ liter per day)	As ready-made juice can be stored for 2(!) years, the necessary amount of 21 liters (which is 42 bottles, 0.5 liter each) may be bought at one time for the entire course of treatment. Now it's time to ask for a wholesale discount ☺

Chapter 11 - Cancer Treatment Shopping List

Onion broth ingredients (Onions: greengrocer's, market place. Broth: grocer's)	
Amount	Notes
Approx. 5 kg (per course of treatment)	Onion (botanical name: Allium cepa L.) for onion broth. You need onions, both approximately the size of a lemon, to boil one a day.
Amount per course of treatment (approx. for 25 liters)	Vegetable bouillon cubes or vegetable broth

Ingredients for broth of bean pods (Note: only for those who cannot tolerate onion broth or have liver or gall bladder diseases) (greengrocer's, market place, herbal medicine and natural product store - Reformhaus, pharmacy, Internet)		
Amount per course of treatment	Name	Notes
Approx. 250 g	Bean pods (botanical name: Phaesoli pericarpium DAC (Phaseoli fructus sine semine)	Fresh, dried or ground bean pods

Hawthorn tincture (herbal medicine and natural product store - Reformhaus, pharmacy, cosmetic store)		
Amount per course of treatment	Name	Notes
Approx. 200 g	(hawthorn, botanical name: Crataegus laevigata Poir.)	To support the heart (pharmacy or herbal medicine and natural product store – Reformhaus)
The alcohol, which the tincture contains, comes in small amounts and is not dangerous.		

Chapter 11 - Cancer Treatment Shopping List

Additional juices
(juices: herbal medicine and natural product store - Reformhaus, cosmetic store; apples: market place)
Sauerkraut juice, lemon juice, freshly-squeezed apple juice, *one mouthful* of which is allowed to be taken from time to time. Buy apples, and never ready-made apple juice. It is not freshly squeezed. Even if the label states the opposite.

Teas for all cancer types		
(pharmacy, herbal medicine and natural product store - Reformhaus, cosmetic store)		
Amount per course of treatment	Horsetail	Equisetum arvense
30 g.	Stinging nettle	Urtica dioica
20 g.	Bird grass (knotgrass)	Polygonum aviculare
15 g.	Sage leaves	Salvia officinali
150 g.	St. John's wort	Hypericum perforatum
110 g.	Peppermint	Mentha piperita
100 g.	Lemon balm	Melissa officinali
100 g.	Marigold	Calendula officinali
100 g.	Cranesbill (herb Robert)	Geranium Robertianum
100 g.	Plantain lance or broadleaf plantain, or their mix 50:50	Plantago lanceolata /
100 g.	Iceland moss	Plantago major
100 g	Lungwort	Pulmonaria officinali
100 g	Ground ivy	Glechoma hederacea
100 g	Mullein	Verbascum densifloru
100 g	Ligusticum mutellina	Meum mutellina → see Chapter 11.

Chapter 11 - Cancer Treatment Shopping List

\multicolumn{3}{c}{**Additional herbal teas for particular cancer types** (pharmacy, herbal medicine and natural product store - Reformhaus, cosmetic store)}		
Amount per course of treatment	Name in English, type of cancer	Botanical name
150 g	Eyebright / eye cancer	Euphrasia rostkoviana
100 g	Willow herb / prostate and testicular cancer	Herba Epilobii parvifloris concis
100 g	Valerian tea / stomach cancer combined with irritable bowel syndrome	Valeriana officinali
250 g	Greater pimpernel / cancer of the palate, lips, tongue, neck lymph nodes and larynx	Pimpinella magna (small P. saxifraga)
100 g	Lemon balm / cerebral tumor	Melissa officinali
150 g	Celandine / skin cancer	Chelidonium majus
100 g	Silvery lady's mantle / breast, ovarian and uterine cancers	Alchemilla, alpina
100 g	Lady's mantle / breast, ovarian and uterine cancers	Alchemilla, vulgaris
100 g	Yellow dead nettle/ breast, ovarian and uterine cancers	Lamium galeobdolon Herb or blossoms
100 g	White dead nettle / breast, ovarian and uterine cancers	Laminum, album
100 g	Wormwood tea / gall bladder, liver and stomach cancer	Artemisia absinthium
100 g	Centaury / stomach cancer	Centaurium erythraea

Chapter 11 - Cancer Treatment Shopping List

Strath Remedies for Recovery (available in Switzerland, Austria and 50 more countries)
No factory-direct sale. On sale in pharmacies, cosmetic and health-related stores, herbal medicine and natural product stores – Reformhaus, organic food shops. Information on distributors – www.bio-strath.ch

Amount per course of treatment (approximately for 2 to 3 months, usually before the treatment and after it):
1 package of 750 ml (50 days, 3x1 coffee spoons a day) or 1 package of 300 tablets (50 days, 2-3 tablets a day); packages of 100 tablets are also available.

PK-Strath herbal yeast (available in Germany)
(Factory-direct sale – see Appendix for address. Alternatively, order from pharmacy)

Amount per course of treatment (approximately for one month, usually before the treatment <u>and</u> after it): 1 double package of 2 x 250 ml or 2 packages of 140 tablets.

Chapter 11 - Cancer Treatment Shopping List

Problems with buying herbal medicines?

Sometimes timely purchase of various medicines for a course of treatment may appear to be a really challenging task. You may face difficulties when trying to buy herbal teas, well-known Ligusticum mutellina or remedies for the recovery period immediately after the treatment.

Can't find Ligusticum mutellina

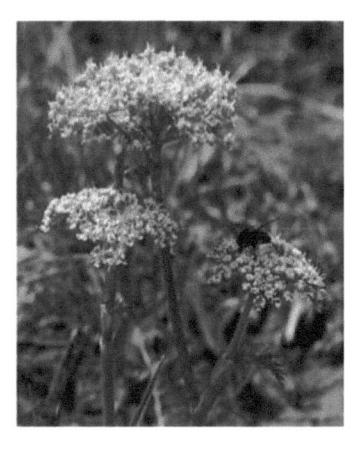

Well, this is the problem which existed during Rudolf Breuss' lifetime. He urged Alpine farmers to grow this herb, which can be found naturally only on mountainsides at a height of 1400 metres and above. But apparently he failed to convince them.

However, the time of fruitless search is now gone: Ligusticum which is popularly styled as "bear root" can be purchased at:

Natural Spinal Care
Owner: Michael Rau
Römerstrasse, 56
74448 Durmersheim
Tel. 07245-937195
Fax 07245-937194
E-mail: info@breuss-dorn-shop.de
Website: www.breuss-dorn-shop.de

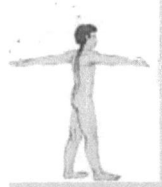

Chapter 11 - Cancer Treatment Shopping List

Natural Spinal Care®

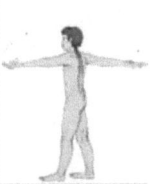

Breuss and Dorn Spinal Care Training Center
And all you need for treatment according to
Rudolf Breuss and Dieter Dorn

We have everything necessary for the treatment process according to Breuss and Dorn, including books, posters, videos, massage oils, care systems and therapy equipment.

Herbal teas, as well as the Breuss vegetable juice for the Breuss fasting therapy, are at your disposal.

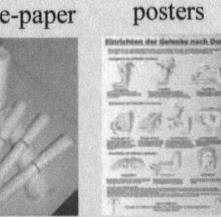

- adjustment valves for spinal alignment
- massage oils
- tissue-paper
- posters
- books about Breuss
- the Breuss herbal tea mix
- the Breuss vegetable juice

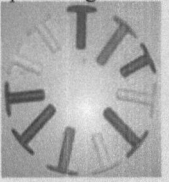

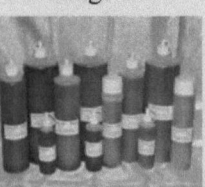

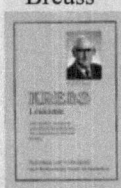

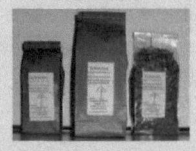

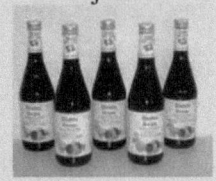

We are always at your service:
Natural Spinal Care®
Römerstrasse, 56
74448 Durmersheim
Tel. 07245-937195
Fax 07245-937194
Check out our online store or schedule of our seminars:
www.breuss-dorn-shop.de www.breuss-dorn-seminare.de

Chapter 11 - Cancer Treatment Shopping List

I would like to express my gratitude to Mr Rau for successfully convincing Alpine farmers to start growing such a useful herb as Ligusticum mutellina.

> **Tip:** <u>Ligusticum mutellina as well as five other herbs</u> is an ingredient for a special tea mix (Chapter 10). According to Breuss, it is <u>not necessary</u> for all six herbs mentioned above to be added to the mix. These words, at least, may comfort the patients trying to find Ligusticum mutellina in vain.
> So, if you do not find Ligusticum mutellina, it won't be a big problem!

Can't find Bio-Strath (Strath)/PK-Strath

In Germany you can purchase PK-Strath herbal yeast either through factory-direct sale (Strath-Labor GmbH, 93093 Donaustauf, Strathstrasse 5-7, Website: www.strath-labor.de, E-mail: strath-labor@t-online.de, Tel.: +40(0)9403 9509 0, Fax: +49(0)9403 9509 20), or in a pharmacy which will order this remedy for you.

In Switzerland, Austria and 50 other countries, Strath remedies for recovery can be found in pharmacies, cosmetic and health-related stores, herbal medicine and natural product stores (Reformhaus), organic food shops. Information on distributors can be found at Bio-Strath AG, CH-8032 Zurich, Mühlebachstrasse, 38. Website: www.bio-strath.ch, E-mail: info@bio-strath.ch, Tel. +41(0)44-2507100

Can't find a herbal tea or vegetable juice

If you are having trouble finding herbal teas and juices, contact Natural Spinal Care, owner: Michael Rau, Römerstrasse, 56, 74448 Durmersheim, Tel. 07245-937195, Fax: 07245-937194, E-mail: info@breuss-dorn-shop.de, Website: www.breuss-dorn-shop.de

CHAPTER 12

The Breuss Total Cancer Treatment Undergoes Clinical Trial

⌘

What I wish for at the time of writing

I would be happy if parts of the oncology report presented below helped the following groups, namely cancer patients, their relatives and medical professionals:

- Representatives of conventional medicine should begin to study The Cure and possibilities related to it in an objective and impartial way.

- Medical doctors, and primarily family doctors, should develop a positive attitude towards their patients' requests for medical supervision when the latter undergo the Breuss Total Cancer Treatment.

- The Breuss Total Cancer Treatment should attract even more interest and attention, with patients more readily accepting the challenges of the 42-day course of treatment.

- Cancer patients and, first and foremost, their kith and kin, should be filled with hope, showing patience and courage, even if the disease has gone so far that no flas of hope can be offered by conventional medicine.

- The trials that are under way should deliver the firs results as soon as possible, in order to provide scientifi evidence of the efficiency and effectiveness of the therapy.

Chapter 12 - The Breuss Total Cancer Treatment Undergoes Clinical Trial

The oncology report by Professor Douwes, MD:
«How reasonable is fasting therapy for treating cancer patients?»
8 terminally ill cancer patients undergo the Breuss Total Cancer Treatment

In December 1982 Rudolf Breuss' sincerest wish for his total cancer treatment "to be tested by conventional medicine" was fulfilled.

In Sonnenberg clinic (a member of the Wicker Group which nowadays comprises 12 emergency and rehabilitation hospitals in Hesse, North Rhine-Westphalia and Thuringia) of Bad Sooden-Allendorf, the Breuss Total Cancer Treatment underwent its first clinical trial. Rudolf Breuss was invited by the owner of the Wicker Clinics to participate personally in the treatment of 8 terminally-ill cancer patients who expressed their desire to undergo the Breuss Total Cancer Treatment.

Friedrich Douwes, MD, Professor, was the medical director of the clinic at that time. He admits being totally ignorant of the Breuss Total Cancer Treatment back then, so he displayed quite a skeptical attitude towards the experiment.

Thus, Rudolf Breuss together with his grandson Walter Margreiter (who publishes books by and about Breuss in Bludenz, Austria), arrived at Bad Sooden-Allendorf to take part in the "experiment" conducted by conventional medical practitioners.

Under Professor Douwes' supervision, in the oncology clinic environment, 8 patients underwent the 42-day course of the Breuss Total Cancer Treatment.

Chapter 12 - The Breuss Total Cancer Treatment Undergoes Clinical Trial

The results appeared to be so positive and surprising for the medical director, Professor Douwes, that he wrote a special "oncology report" on this experience. The report, which was entitled "How reasonable is fasting therapy for treating cancer patients?", was published in a specialized "Journal of Cancer Research and Clinical Oncology".

As the above-mentioned report can greatly contribute to the trustworthiness of the beneficial effect displayed by the Breuss Total Cancer Treatment, and due to the fact that it was written by a representative of conventional medicine, I would like to present some extracts from this document here. I am citing the report word for word, giving in brackets my own commentaries marked as "Ed.". The title and source of this report can be found in References of the "Oncology" chapter.

«Pilot study of the 42-day vegetable juice treatment of 8 terminally ill cancer patients»

Every oncologist during their lifetime meets patients whose advanced disease does not leave any hope for being treated by conventional methods. Unfortunately, those situations happen quite often. When medical doctors appear to be helpless, the patients and their kith and kin try to fall back on alternative medical method of treatment. And the question that often arises is why not act in the best interests of the patients and conduct such an alternative treatment in clinic environment? This would also give an opportunity to check how effective these alternative methods are.

From the patients we have heard about Rudolf Breuss, an Austrian naturopath, who claimed to have cured many cancer patients, including those with advanced-stage cancer, with his 42-day vegetable juice treatment. After gathering all the available information on this method of treatment (scientific publications on it do not exist), and urged by the desire of our 8 patients to undergo this 42-day course of fasting therapy

Chapter 12 - The Breuss Total Cancer Treatment Undergoes Clinical Trial

and juice diet, we agreed to give it a try even though there were solid grounds for having doubts and concerns. In carrying it out, we pursued the following two goals:

a) if the patient has been undergoing such a treatment, it is better to do it under the supervision of a medical doctor who in a timely manner can recognize and eliminate all possible risks; and

b) to carry out critical evaluation of this method of treatment in order to determine its effectiveness or ineffectiveness.

Procedure

Before the start of the therapy, all its participants had been warned of the possible risks.
They all expressed their written consent to conducting such an experiment and participating in it.

All patients had metastatic cancerous tumors of various localisations, wherein conventional treatment methods were either exhausted or inapplicable.

Before the experiment began, all the patients were thoroughly examined and the data were recorded.

The therapy involved a 42-day fast when the patients did not eat solid food drank only half a liter to one liter of vegetable juice on a daily basis made from a mix of red beet (3/5), carrot (1/5), celery (1/5), as well as a small amount of radish and potato juice, enriched with whey[18] (the Breuss juice by Biotta).

Besides "the Breuss juice", each day the patients had two bowls of

---

18) When professor Douwes mentions "whey" here, it is not a whey in the ordinary sense of the word, but a substance added to the Biotta ready-made vegetable juice for its shelf stability

Chapter 12 - The Breuss Total Cancer Treatment Undergoes Clinical Trial

vegetable salt-free broth, and approximately 2 liters of liquid in the form of various herbal teas (sage, cranesbill, horsetail, stinging nettle, St. John's wort, etc.).

Virtually no medication was administered to the patients, though they still received painkillers. Besides, the patients underwent regular balneological and physical procedures (Ed.: i.e., **therapy swimming pool, massages, mud wraps, electrotherapy**), *and were engaged in physical activities.*

Furthermore, the patients had three group sessions a day; twice a week the group sessions were led by our psychologists.

Medical supervision

The patients were under constant medical supervision, which was carried out via regular blood and urine tests. Besides the control of general indicators, such as ESR, complete blood count, liver and kidneys function tests, special attention was paid to nitrogen metabolism, electrolytes and blood gases. The patients were weighed three times a day.

Results

Table 7 (Ed.: In the original report, see References) *generalizes the patients' data, as well as the therapy results. It is worth mentioning that after the end of the 42-day fasting therapy, which was strictly adhered to by all the patients, two cases displayed complete remission, namely, a patient with stage IVb Hodgkin lymphoma (lymphogranuloma) and another patient with visceral metastatic mamma carcinoma.* (Ed.: **complete remission means the absence of signs and symptoms of the disease in the course of an imaging examination over the course of 6 months**).

Chapter 12 - The Breuss Total Cancer Treatment Undergoes Clinical Trial

Casuistics (Ed.: personal case study reports).

H.H. (53 years old), stage IVb Hodgkin lymphoma (Ed.: lymphoid cancer): *Manifestations of Hodgkin lymphoma were located mainly in mediastinum* (Ed.: vertical septum of the thoracic cavity surrounded by connective tissue) *and in spleen. Besides, the patient had acute B-symptoms such as anemia, fever and night sweats. The previous therapy involved COPP chemotherapy regimen* (Ed.: chemotherapy consisting of four drugs), *as well as ABVD chemotherapy regimen* (Ed.: chemotherapy consisting of four other drugs). *Histologically* (Ed.: concerning tissues taken for examination), *it is a mixed cell type. The B-symptoms were gone. As early as in the process of fasting therapy and consumption of vegetable juice. Mediastinal lymph nodes shrank. 11 months after this uncommon therapy* (Ed.: the Breuss Total Cancer Treatment), *the patient still has none of the symptoms mentioned above. A recent computed tomography has not identified any signs of pathological lymphoma* (Ed.: pathological lymph node enlargement).

E. Y. (59 years old), metastatic mamma carcinoma (Ed.: metastatic breast cancer): *another <u>complete remission</u> was observed in the case of metastatic mamma carcinoma. It was mainly visceral metastasis of the the left lung. Trial treatment with tamoxifen and medroxyprogesterone acetate was not successful. In the process of fasting therapy, the patient displayed a drop in the slightly increased oncofetal antigen indicators, and her solitary coin lesions slowly shrank in size up to their almost complete disappearance. It was only recently that the lung manifestation* (Ed.: suspected lung problem) *has appeared again. Tests also show slightly increased values of oncomarkers.*

H.H. (63 years old), metastatic carcinoma of the prostate (Ed.: metastatic prostate cancer): *in this case of bone locoregional visceral metastatic carcinoma of the prostate, we managed to achieve <u>partial remission</u>. Hormone therapy, as well as estramustine (estracyt) treatment* (Ed.: hormone and chemotherapy) *were exhausted.*

Chapter 12 - The Breuss Total Cancer Treatment Undergoes Clinical Trial

In the process of fasting therapy, the pain was significantly relieved; besides, a temporary reduction in prostate acid phosphatase (Ed.: **oncomarker**) *was observed. X-ray diagnosis did not identify any tendencies for bone healing. After the treatment the patient felt well and had no complaints for almost 6 months. However, in the 7th month after the therapy, he died of cerebral metastasis* (Ed.: **cerebral tumor**).

E.H. (55 years old), metastatic lung adenocarcinoma (Ed.: **tumor that develops in glandular tissues**): *one more <u>partial remission</u> with slight recurrence of liver metastasis, as well as that of pulmonary* (Ed.: **lung**) *foci was achieved in the case of metastatic lung adenocarcinoma. Besides a positive effect on the tumor, the patient displayed an obvious improvement in her performance status and general state of health. One more notable thing was that the process of treatment put an end to the patient's pain and significantly reduced her old cough.*

G.L., (64 years old), metastatic colon carcinoma (Ed.: **colon cancer**): *this patient with metastatic colon carcinoma had previously been treated with phthoruracilum and nitrosourea, with no more opportunity to be treated with chemotherapy. In the process of fasting therapy, the growth of his tumor temporarily discontinued and was accompanied by a reduction in oncomarker levels. However, thereupon his tumor slowly resumed its growth and it is continuing to grow at the present moment. The patient also displayed improvements in his overall health. His Karnofsky Performance Scale Index* (Ed.: **Karnofsky Performance Scale Index allows to see a patient's performance status, to assess whether they are able to care for personal needs or require special assistance with their needs**) *which constituted 50% at the beginning of the course of treatment, grew to 90% after the therapy. We considered this very case to be the most indicative and selected it for presentation in Fig.1 (in the original report).*

Two patients (G.E., 66 years old and E.Y., 40 years old), with extensive incurable mamma carcinomas (Ed.: **breast cancer**): *for these two*

Chapter 12 - The Breuss Total Cancer Treatment Undergoes Clinical Trial

patients, the course of treatment produced no results. One of them, E.Y., with symptoms of high intracranial pressure, died in the course of treatment due to the after-effects of cerebral metastasis. Another patient (G.E.) died immediately after the course of treatment. At the same time, in the process of treatment both patients had reported subjective improvements in overall health due to significantly relieved pains. Besides, in the process of fasting therapy, the patients' extensive lymphedemas caused by a tumor (Ed.: meaning **visible and palpable fluid collection**) *shrank, so in this context the pain was almost gone. Furthermore, these patients readily participated in group sessions guided by psychologists and died at peace with themselves and the world around them.*

B.Sh. (69 years old), pancreas carcinoma (Ed.: **Pancreatic cancer**)*: in this case of pancreas carcinoma, a few weeks after the fasting therapy, the patient died in cachexia* (Ed.: **cachexia is an ultimate loss of body mass. In medicine, it is represented by the body mass index below 18**)*. Similar to the case above, she did not feel pain in the process of treatment and seemed to be more even-minded and calm than before. Partial intestinal obstructions* (Ed.: **intestinal pseudo-obstruction**) *which before the treatment course had forced us to intervene therapeutically, were not observed in the process of fasting therapy, but they recurred immediately after the adaptation* (Ed.: **adjusting to**) *to normal nutrition.*

Conclusions

To sum up, we may point out that

- *During the 42-day fasting therapy together with the juice diet 8 patients felt significantly better than was expected.*
- *During this period they remained active except for those patients who had been bedridden before the treatment started.*
- *After the treatment, most patients displayed considerable improvements in their state of health, and in the course of three*

Chapter 12 - The Breuss Total Cancer Treatment Undergoes Clinical Trial

months they managed to reach higher values of the Karnofsky index.

- During the treatment period the weight loss averaged 11.7 kg (the average value was 11.4 kg). It varied from 8.9 to 15.6 kg. The biggest weight loss was observed in overweight patients, while that of others tended towards lower values.
- Four weeks following the treatment most patients gained their original weight.
- Further complications did not arise. Lab. values did not in general undergo essential changes or deviations. That is why they are not discussed here. Only in one case was there an increase in uric acid, which required medication therapy.

Discussion

The 42-day fasting therapy with simultaneous adherence to a juice diet did not worsen the condition of any patient. One patient's death in the process of treatment was not linked to the treatment itself, but to cerebral metastasis she had developed before the therapy started, so by the start of the treatment course her life expectancy was less than three months.

The same is true of two other patients who died immediately after the fasting therapy, having in general benefited from it. Most importantly, they no longer suffered from pain and could go without painkillers, which had a positive impact on their state of mind.

Five remaining patients, considering the dynamics of their diseases, also benefited from participating in this course of treatment. The condition of one patient did not undergo significant changes, while two other patients displayed temporary partial remission, and two other patients had complete remission.

Chapter 12 - The Breuss Total Cancer Treatment Undergoes Clinical Trial

Friedrich Douwes, MD, professor, Sonnenberg Clinic

– This is the end of the extract from the oncology report –

(Ed.) *As a reader of the "Oncology Report", I can state that the overall health of only six out of eight patients pronounced incurable by conventional medicine allowed them to undergo The Cure, and two of them, that is one third, **regained their health**. And for these patients cured of cancer this may be called "a gift from above", or from Rudolf Breuss and his juice treatment.*

Feedback from conventional medical community

Veronica Karstens, MD, in her scientific paper "Empirical cancer diagnosis and therapy", among other issues also mentions

Congress of the German Society for Oncology, held on 5.11.1983 in Baden-Baden

citing Dr. Douwes, MD, professor, who presented a report on his pilot project.

Let me cite Dr. Karstens verbatim:

- *Eight hopeless cancer patients with metastatic spread, for whom all possible methods of treatment proved useless, expressed their desire to undergo the Breuss fasting therapy.*
- *The result appeared to be stunning: in as little as four days the patients stopped suffering from pain and improved their overall health.*
- *After the end of treatment two patients were clinically cured of metastasis and tumors, and in four patients, tumors and metastasis shrank.*

Chapter 12 - The Breuss Total Cancer Treatment Undergoes Clinical Trial

- *Only two patients died* (Ed.: I would like to add that these patients were bedridden that is why they could hardly undergo the treatment).

Assessment of results

Dr. Douwes, MD, Professor, addressing the Congress, assessed the results as follows:

«*If we consider the Breuss fasting therapy as a kind of* **medication***, we have to admit that it is absolutely safe and quite effective for terminal cancer, as it was beneficial for 75% of cancer patients*».

Then he added:
«*Such medication should be used* **at the beginning of the treatment**, *rather than at its end, after radical methods* (Ed.: that is surgery, irradiation and chemotherapy) *weaken the patient's immune system*».

No comment, I would say.

Chapter 12 - The Breuss Total Cancer Treatment Undergoes Clinical Trial

There is some progress in the case!
Current state of affairs

«*I would be very happy if my Total Cancer Treatment could be improved by combining it with other successful methods of cancer treatment*», Rudolf Breuss writes in his classical book «Natural Treatment of Cancer, Leukemia and Other Seemingly Incurable Diseases».

Elsewhere in the book he writes, «*Finally I would like to earnestly ask all reputable scientists to test my achievements scientifically..., to be with me in helping the afflicted, instead of being against me for the only reason of my not being a medical professional*».

This naturopath's wish has not been granted yet. However, I am falling under the impression that – at last! – there is some progress in the case.

On the basis of their own positive experience of tumor treatment, a group of traditional medical scientists and naturopathic healers of various specializations is planning to study the Breuss Total Cancer Treatment.

Firstly, in the process of two investigations it is planned to apply scientific methods to analyzing the impact area and mode of action of this therapy. Hopefully, this efficient «empirical» method will attract due attention and might even get further development based on recent medical breakthroughs.

Chapter 12 - The Breuss Total Cancer Treatment Undergoes Clinical Trial

My possible contribution will be made with great pleasure and interest. Nowadays, I am busy with processing and generalizing the formularies I got to gather information on the Breuss Total Cancer Treatment for evaluation by professionals and experts. However, as one man is no man, I am not sure whether it will be possible to make real progress in the near future.

Such research is time-consuming and very costly. Until there is a powerful expert group for conducting these types of research, and an affluent sponsor to support them, there is hardly any hope for real success.

I consider the forms I have collected to be an essential support for conducting the investigations as they are a sort of database for cancer patients (anonymous data) and their cancer types were successfully cured with the help of the Breuss Total Cancer Treatment.

It would be highly desirable to create a database for patients cured of cancer who would agree to give advice, references and recommendations to other patients willing to receive them.

♒

CHAPTER 13
CURRENT CANCER STATISTICS

⌘

New Cancer Cases

New Cancer Cases Worldwide

Here are some terrifying updated figures[19] on recent cancer incidence, that is, as of **2008** (these are the latest statistics)

- Approximately 12.7 million new cases of cancer were diagnosed worldwide,
- There are an estimated 22 million people living with cancer around the world,
- 7.6 million people died of cancer globally.

Experts estimate that in **2030**

- Approximately 26 million people a year will develop cancer worldwide, an increase of 120%.
- 17 million people will die of cancer worldwide, an increase of 225%!

So we are in for some rough times ahead!
What about the chances for a cure?

Today, an average of some 30% of cancer patients are cured of their disease by conventional medicine. In other words:

---

19)   Partly "contradictory" figures in the following summary of the atest and most important tendencies are due to differences in sources, data acquisition methods, estimates and, possibly, incomplete cancer registration.

to date, seven out of every ten cancer patients die!

Cancer is still primarily treated symptomatically, through, chemotherapy, hormonal and radiation therapies, while the real causes of this disease are ignored.

Just as before, far little attention is paid to natural methods of preventing and treating cancer, so that healthy eating and a balanced lifestyle in this regard are largely neglected.

The world is now confronted with a new reality: an increasing number of cancer patients and deaths caused by malignant diseases. This is a consequence of the increasing life expectancy seen throughout the world.

"This year, cancer will replace cardiovascular disease as 'the number one killer'. And *"Cancer case has doubled over the last 30 years",* David J. Kerr, the President of the European Society for Medical Oncology (ESMO) warned, speaking at the European ESMO Congress in Milan on October 12, 2010.

New Cancer Cases in Germany

Here are the figures on recent cancer incidence:
Every year

- 450,000 people develop cancer in Germany,
- 216,000 people die of cancer.

Experts estimate that by 2050 the number of cancer cases will increase by 30%.

The reason: the population is aging, and cancer is a disease that mainly affects elderly people.

Chapter 13 - Current Cancer Statistics

Most Common Cancers in Males

With some 64, 370 new cases diagnosed in Germany each year, prostate cancer is currently the most common cancer type in males. The primary reason for this is the growing number of elderly men. The average age for the illness is around 69 years. The second most common cancer type in males is colorectal cancer, with about 39, 410 newly- diagnosed cases annually. Lung cancer, with some 35, 150 annually diagnosed cases in men is in third place[20].

Most Common Cancers in Females

Breast cancer is the most common cancer among women. In Germany, approximately 59, 510 women are diagnosed with it each year. The average age for the illness is around 64 years. Forty per cent of the women affected are under 60. The second most common cancer type in women is colorectal cancer, with about 33, 620 new cases every year. Lung cancer is third among women – about 15, 180 new cases annually. The reason behind it is the increasing number of female smokers[19]

Childhood Cancers

Each year in Germany, around 1, 800 children and adolescents under the age of 15 develop cancer. This number has been consistent for many years. Today, the chances of cure are at 80%. Malignant neoplasms are still the second leading cause of mortality among children. The most common childhood cancers are leukemia (blood cancer), brain and spinal cord tumors, and cancer of the lymph nodes.[19]

---

20) German Cancer Aid, http://www.krebshilfe.de/krebszahlen.html
As of March 2010

Children and the Breuss treatment: generally, children under 10 should not fast. In any case, before a child begins fasting, you should consult your family doctor or a doctor specializing in fasting.

CANCER Diagnosis

Currently there are almost 1.5 million tumor patients in Germany in whom the disease was diagnosed within the last 5 years.

According to experts, in the current year (2010), the number of people diagnosed with cancer will also grow. Most commonly, men fall ill with prostate cancer, and women – with breast cancer.

At the opening of the 29th German Cancer Congress in Berlin, experts of the Robert Koch Institute (RKI) put forward a worrying prognosis:

In 2010, a new cancer will be diagnosed almost every minute. Malignant tumors will be found in about 450, 000 people.

Since 1990, the number of new cancer cases in Germany has increased by nearly 30%. At the same time, these cases show a considerable gender difference: for men this number has increased by 45%, and for women by 14%. However, the main reason for this is that the present generations of men live much longer than pre-war generations.

The President of German Cancer Aid, Harald zur Hausen, expects that by the year 2030, the number of cancer cases in Germany will increase by 30%.

Chapter 13 - Current Cancer Statistics

"We have to face the fact that by the year 2030, 580,000 cancer cases will be diagnosed each year – almost one third more than now", the Nobel Laureate for Medicine said in an interview. The growing tendency is explained by people living increasingly longer.

He called for preventive measures: *"Nowadays, we know: around two thirds of all cancer cases are the result of our lifestyle"*. *"Abstinence from smoking, reduced alcohol consumption, physical activity»*, continued the President of the German Cancer Aid, *"protection against UV radiation, as well as prevention of viral infections can dramatically reduce cancer risks."*

Cancer diagnosis should not be perceived as a verdict, Mr. zur Hausen emphasized.

Chapter 13 - Current Cancer Statistics

Cancer Diagnosis

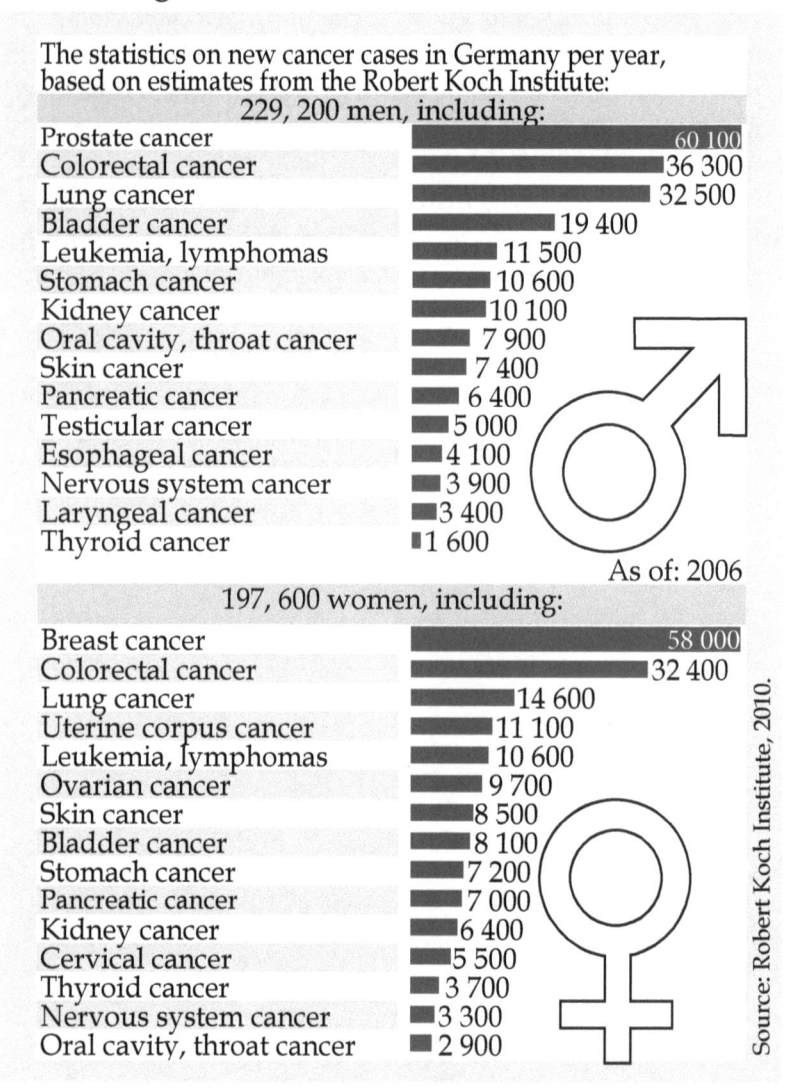

The statistics on new cancer cases in Germany per year, based on estimates from the Robert Koch Institute:

229,200 men, including:

Prostate cancer	60 100
Colorectal cancer	36 300
Lung cancer	32 500
Bladder cancer	19 400
Leukemia, lymphomas	11 500
Stomach cancer	10 600
Kidney cancer	10 100
Oral cavity, throat cancer	7 900
Skin cancer	7 400
Pancreatic cancer	6 400
Testicular cancer	5 000
Esophageal cancer	4 100
Nervous system cancer	3 900
Laryngeal cancer	3 400
Thyroid cancer	1 600

As of: 2006

197,600 women, including:

Breast cancer	58 000
Colorectal cancer	32 400
Lung cancer	14 600
Uterine corpus cancer	11 100
Leukemia, lymphomas	10 600
Ovarian cancer	9 700
Skin cancer	8 500
Bladder cancer	8 100
Stomach cancer	7 200
Pancreatic cancer	7 000
Kidney cancer	6 400
Cervical cancer	5 500
Thyroid cancer	3 700
Nervous system cancer	3 300
Oral cavity, throat cancer	2 900

Source: Robert Koch Institute, 2010.

Estimated number of newly detected cancer cases by cancer type and sex (Source: Robert Koch Institute, 2010)

Chapter 13 - Current Cancer Statistics

Prostate Cancer, Scourge among Men

Nowadays, with some 48,650 new cases diagnosed in Germany every year, prostate cancer is the most common cancer type among men. The main reason for that is the growing number of older men. The average age for the illness is around 71 years. At the same time, 85% of all men over 65 develop prostate cancer[21]. Many of those affected often know nothing about their cancer because they do not undergo preventive cancer screening!

Prostate cancer is the sixth most common cancer in the world. It is the third most common cancer among men worldwide. In Europe (including Germany!), North America and in parts of Africa it is the most common cancer type. It is estimated that in 2010, prostate cancer will be the major cause of death[21].

The age of patients is a crucial factor in prostate cancer statistics. More than 80% of all men diagnosed with prostate cancer are over 60 . For a person aged 50 to 85, the chance of developing prostate cancer increases by fortyfold[22].

According to law, every man from the age of 45 is entitled to a free annual preventive cancer screening for early detection of cancer. De facto, however, only 15% of all men take advantage of this opportunity.

Preventive Cancer Screening

Most common screening methods range from rectal examination (palpation) and transrectal ultrasonography to the PSA (prostate-specific antigen) test (see p. 123). To select

---

21)   Dr. med. N.M. Blumstein, University Hospital Ulm, "Imaging prostate cancer with PET", BPS Journal, an information medium for prostate cancer patients and their relatives, № 2, 2003.
22)   German Cancer Society, "Prostate cancer – causes and risk factors", www.krebsgesellschaft.de/db_prostatakrebs_ursache_und_risikofaktoren,4281.html

Chapter 13 - Current Cancer Statistics

the most effective method, you should discuss the issue with your doctor. In my case, prostate cancer was diagnosed during a routine checkup using methods one and three. Therefore, my personal experience is shaped by my fight against this particular cancer type. However, according to Rudolf Breuss, his treatment can be used for all cancer types (see Chapter 4, Differentiated Treatment for Various Cancer Types), so the approach described in this book can be applied to any other cancer type, with no major adjustments.

Breast Cancer, Scourge among Women

In women aged 40 to 50, breast cancer (mamma carcinoma) is the major cause of death. In Germany, 53 women die of this disease each day, which means around 20, 000 women per year. Around 46,000 women are diagnosed with breast cancer every single year. Many women who die of breast cancer are under 40. Breast cancer is by far the most common cancer among women. Almost one in ten women will develop this kind of tumor in their lifetime[23].

In Germany, breast cancer accounts for 40% of all new cancer incidences; it is the most common cancer among women. According to the Robert Koch Institute, every year around **55,100** women in Germany develop mamma carcinoma, with 23,200 of them being under the age of 60 at the time of diagnosis.

The risk of contracting this disease increases gradually after the fourth decade of life. The average age for the illness is a little over 62 years[24].

---

23) WDR channel, WDRPunkt Dortmund "Health" program, 15.2.2005, www.wdr.de/studio/dortmund/wpunkt/service/gesundheit/150205_brustkrebs.html
24) Gynecologists in the Net, Professional Association of Gynecologists, www.frauen-aerzte-im-netz.de/de_allgemeine-haeufigkeit_365.html

Chapter 13 - Current Cancer Statistics

In the USA, the incidence of breast cancer is six times higher, and in Germany – nearly five times higher than in Japan. When Japanese women emigrated to the USA, their risk of breast cancer does not significantly increase. However, the risk of developing breast cancer for their daughters and especially granddaughters approaches the high risk of breast cancer for American women. In Europe, the highest breast cancer incidence rates are registered in the Netherlands, Denmark, Finland and Sweden. As for Germany, with its breast cancer incidence rates it occupies a middle position among European countries. The lowest disease rates are found in the Southern European countries, namely Spain, Greece and Portugal[25].

There is no clear explanation for these regional differences. Researchers believe that this is primarily due to giving birth to the first child at an older age, childlessness, earlier menarche (first menstrual period) or later menopause (physiological end of menstrual periods)[25].

In various studies researchers also point to the connection with nutritional habits – in particular, high-calorie nutrition – and high consumption of alcohol[25].

Early Cancer Screening

Preventive breast cancer screening is a component of statutory cancer screening procedures for women over 30. The costs of this preventive screening are covered by public healthcare funds.

Mammography (an x-ray examination of mammary glands) is an essential component of early detection of cancer and the foundation of mass breast cancer screening. Germany

---
25) German Cancer Society, New Cancer Cases in Women, www.krebsgesellschaft.de/krebshaeufigkeit.11267.htm

Chapter 13 - Current Cancer Statistics

is currently developing a quality-assured mammography screening program based on the "European Guidelines for Quality Assurance in Mammography Screening".

By the end of 2007, a total of 89 mammography devices were planned to be operational throughout Germany. In some regions, mammography screening is already available for the target group (women aged 50 to 69)[26].

Mammography is a **crucial** examination used for detecting any changes in breast tissue. In addition to mammography, it may be desirable to make an ultrasound scan. However, the final diagnosis cannot be made on the basis of these imaging techniques only, without examining tissue samples (biopsy) taken from an area of concern. A biopsy can also be helpful for determining the aggressiveness of the tumor or hormone binding sites. Both factors influence therapy. In addition, a tissue sample is analyzed to assess the so-called HER2 receptors (human epidermal growth factor receptor 2) – the receptors stimulating healthy mammary gland cells to grow, split and recover[26].

The more HER2 receptors that are produced by a mammary gland cell, the more growth signals it receives. The cell splits itself again and again, and the tumor continues to grow[27].

About 25%-30% of all women with breast cancer display high levels of HER2 receptors in the epithelium of the mammary gland. It has been discovered that high levels of HER2 receptors are often linked to an unfavourable and more aggressive tumor development.

In such cases it may make sense to block HER2 receptors with an antibody, thereby removing growth stimulation27.

26) DKV Deutsche Krankenversicherung AG, Cologne
27) krebs-aktuell.de,
http://www.gesundheit-aktuell.de/krebs-aktuell/informationen-ueber-krebs/archive/2006.html

Chapter 13 - Current Cancer Statistics

Colorectal Cancer, Scourge among Men and Women

Colorectal cancer is the second most common cancer among both sexes. According to the Robert Koch Institute, around 35,000 men and the same number of women in Germany contract this cancer type every year.

The death rate from colorectal cancer has been steadily decreasing since the mid-1970s. Nevertheless, it remains the second major cause of death from cancer[28].

Colorectal cancer develops predominantly after the age of 50. The average age for patients diagnosed with colorectal cancer is 69 for men, and for women it is substantially higher – 75. Based on current estimates, about 6% of the population, i.e. almost 5 million people in Germany, run the risk of developing colorectal cancer at some point in their lives[28].

Early Cancer Screening

For both men and women over 50, colorectal cancer screening is an **important** part of early detection of cancer. A current study proves the effectiveness of this procedure[29].

The study evaluated 110, 000 screening colonoscopies. This is one third of all ambulatory examinations conducted in Germany from October 2003 to July 2005.

---

28)   German Cancer Society, www.krebsgesellschaft.de/darmkrebs_definition_haeufigkeit,45178.ht
29)   A. Sieg and A. Theilmeier: Results of Colonoscopy Screening 2005; German Medical Weekly, 2006; 131 (8): p. 379-383.

Chapter 13 - Current Cancer Statistics

Contributing to the speed with which the data were analysed, 280 GP surgeries uploaded their records to the internet database. The results published in the German Medical Weekly suggest the effectiveness of colonoscopy: one out of five persons over 55 – from this age onwards the examination is recommended every ten years – had colon polyps.

These are benign growths which can eventually lead to colorectal cancer. Around 30% of these polyps were so far advanced that the growth could become cancerous at any time.[29]

Most polyps could be immediately removed during colonoscopy. The investigators see it as a significant advantage of the procedure, since according to studies by American scientists, removing polyps reduces the incidence of colorectal cancer by nearly 90%.[29]

Chapter 13 - Current Cancer Statistics

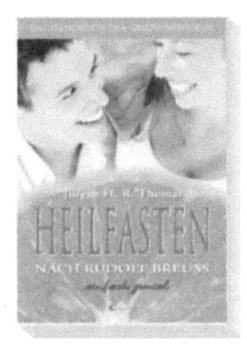

Jürgen H.R. Thomar

Rudolf Breuss Fasting Therapy – Simply Ingenious
GUIDE TO CANCER TREATMENT
DIE SILBERSCHNUR Publishing House, 2007
Detailed tips on the fasting cure – including the post-treatment period!
This book shows you how you should change your life, either before or after the Breuss treatment. Here you will find all the necessary details.
The book is an ideal supplement to books on treatment procedures.

A5, 176 pages, paperback
€ (Germany) 14,90; (Austria) 15,40; CHF 26,80
ISBN 978-3-89845-191-8

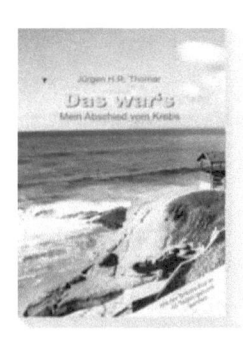

Jürgen H.R. Thomar

That Was It
My Farewell from Cancer
Pocketbook
Amazon, March 2015
This book will tell you how I lived, how I found my way to the Breuss cure, how I fought against cancer and won this fight. It will also provide important details on the basics of this method, which you may find helpful in starting your own treatment.

This book is designed to pave the way to cure for cancer patients.
A5, 157 pages, paperback
€ (France/Germany/Austria) 13,70
ISBN 978-150 841 6234

CHAPTER 14

For the Benefit of the People

⌘

Quo Vadis[30], cancer treatment

The growths of the world's population, medical progress and many other factors have contributed to the fact that over the last few years the healthcare sector has become an independent industry with high growth rates.

In particular, cancer treatment based on modern drugs and medical equipment represents a significant market, so that some branches of the healthcare sector may be interested in increased sales revenues due to of high cancer rates. Conventional cancer treatment can easily cost between 100,000 and 200,000 Euros and in many cases this amount will not be sufficient.

Naturally, the research and development of cancer drugs are very cost intensive; the main issue, however, is whether the optimization of shareholder value (shareholders' income) in the field of cancer medicine should come so far to the fore. Should this important, life-saving cancer treatment be so expensive? Won't it even destroy, in the long run, our healthcare system?

Can't or even mustn't the wish that Rudolf Breuss once expressed, *"I would be very happy if my cancer treatment could*

---

[30] Quo vadis? is a Latin phrase meaning, "Where are you going?" In daily use this phrase is often used in the sense, "Where shall we end up?" or "What will all this come to?"

be improved by combining with other successful methods of cancer treatment"*, help to minimize the costs that are predominantly borne by society?

Perhaps it is time for the politicians in charge of the healthcare system, doctors and health insurance providers, to assess the extent to which we should follow the advice of Prof. Dr. Douwes and apply "The Cure" *at the very beginning* of the therapy, thus giving many cancer patients hope of recovery?

Fasting cancer treatment starts the therapy!

Back in spring 1983, Prof. Dr. Douwes, after assessing the results of the Breuss cancer treatment received from a clinical trial, brought forward the idea that it would be reasonable to conduct the Breuss treatment <u>at the beginning</u> of cancer therapy. And only then, if the treatment fails, one should start – or resume - conventional medical treatment (radiotherapy, surgery, chemotherapy).

Rudolf Breuss also advocated this approach and, from my own experience, I would like to completely associate myself with it.

If the patient's condition allows "The Cure" then it would, on the one hand, spare many patients from a great deal of burdensome diagnostics and therapies and, on the other hand, significantly lighten the load on our health insurance providers

40% of all cancer cases can be prevented!

Changes in lifestyle, improved prevention and early detection methods **can prevent up to 40% of all cancer cases**, the WHO

Regional Office for Europe said on the occasion of World Cancer Day in 2010.

People, themselves, can substantially reduce their cancer risks by avoiding risk factors (such as tobacco use, heavy alcohol consumption, excessive sun exposure and obesity) and adopting healthier lifestyles.

As cancer incidence rates continue to rise, **governments** have to play a crucial role in raising awareness and introducing comprehensive early detection measures.

"Well-conceived and effective national cancer control programs are essential in fighting cancer and improving the lives of cancer patients", says Zsuzsanna Jakab, the WHO Regional Director for Europe. *" We urge all governments to rigorously implement the four basic components of cancer control – prevention, early detection, diagnosis and treatment"* .

Will our **governments** follow the advice of the WHO, for the benefit of the people, so that they do not become cancer patients?

The role of the patient

For large segments of the population, the understanding of role allocation between the patient and the doctor has probably been molded for decades, if not for centuries. The doctor, through his long and comprehensive training and social status, is credited with the power to restore the patient's health by using various methods and drugs.
For the patient it is, on the one hand, convenient as responsibility is handed over. On the other hand, a feeling

Chapter 14 - FOR THE BENEFIT OF THE PEOPLE

of dependency and incapacitation emerges. The awareness of how much a person can do for his or her own recovery has changed dramatically. Likewise, the willingness to spare time and effort for personal health has declined.

On the other hand, the patient has become more critical and enlightened. He or she no longer unconditionally relies on the health system, trying instead to stay constantly informed about diseases and therapies.
Patients no longer blindly trust their doctor or alternative practitioner. They want to be "convinced" that the measures offered to them are exactly what they need. If the physician fails to do so, the "enlightened patients" will be looking, more actively than ever before, for the right - from their point of view - solution.

If the patients see the Breuss treatment as a chance to get healthy again, they should realize that fasting 42 days is not a simple and convenient route. It calls for considerable courage, determination and perseverance if they wish to follow this route.

Numerous patients, who, in the meantime, have recovered from cancer thanks to the Breuss treatment, demonstrate that the effort is worth it.

CHAPTER 15

I Have a Vision

⌘

May wishes come true

May all the participants in the healthcare system, from doctors and the medical industry to individual patients, become ever more aware that the focus of all considerations and efforts is the human being as a harmonious creature.

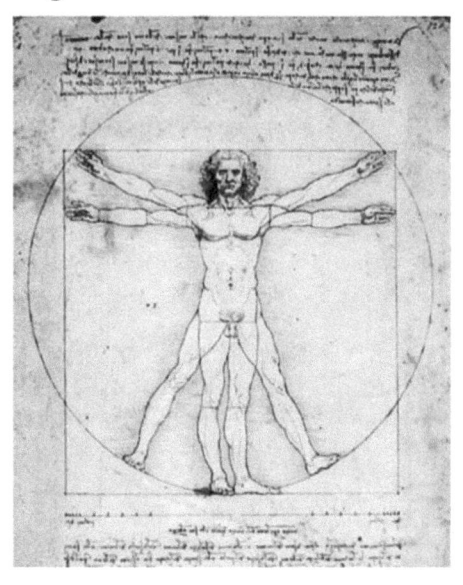

May patients become aware of their own vital power, in harmony with all medical disciplines contribute, to the best of their knowledge and belief, to the recovery of the patient.

Chapter 15 - I Have a Vision

May Rudolf Breuss' cordial request for scientific verification of his successes in discovering cancer treatment become a reality.

May this vision be fulfilled within my lifetime, because Rudolf Breuss, whom we owe the successful treatment of cancer through his vegetable juice diet, will unfortunately never see his dream come true.

May one day physicians, having considered available therapeutic possibilities:

- Breuss treatment,
- Surgery,
- Radiotherapy,
- Chemotherapy,
- Hormone therapy,

select a therapy which is tailored to the patient's individual needs and his or her specific disease. For the patient's benefit

As a reminder: on November 5, 1983, the well-known oncologist Prof. Dr. Friedrich Douwes, addressing the Congress of the German Society for Oncology in Baden-Baden, shared the impressions which he gained from the clinical trial of the Breuss juice fasting cancer treatment (see Chapter 12).

He assessed the results in the following way: *"If we consider the Breuss fasting therapy as a kind of **medication**, we have to admit that it is absolutely safe and quite effective for terminal cancer, as it was beneficial for 75% of cancer patients"*.

Chapter 15 - I Have a Vision

He added, *"Such medication should be used at the beginning of the treatment, rather than at its end, after radical methods weaken the patient's immune system".*

May this assessment of the Breuss cancer treatment, made by Prof. Douwes, motivate as many practitioners of conventional medicine as possible to investigate, objectively and impartially, the Breuss method and the possibilities it offers to their cancer patients.

Dear readers, now, at the end of my book, I would like to express my personal wish:

I wish, for the good of all cancer patients who want to participate in shared decision- making, that your doctor would, on his own initiative, right after you are diagnosed with cancer:

- Advise you as a first step – and at your earliest convenience – to undergo the Breuss cancer treatment;
- Furthermore, to ensure successful recovery, offer you his medical supervision.

Jürgen H.R. Thomar

Chapter 15 - I Have a Vision

APPENDIX 1

DAILY SCHEDULE

When undergoing the course of cancer treatment, nobody needs to get up at 6 o'clock or earlier, unless this is a demand of the job.

The schedule specified below is a tentative one. The left-hand column indicates my time, while the right-hand column is reserved for your time. You can start your day at, let's say, no earlier than 9 or no later than 4:30 am, rescheduling all the time indicators below by 3 hours backwards, or by 1.5 hours forward. Times and sequences are the same for each day; however, discontinue using kidney tea starting from day 22.

If you have (or wish) to go to work during the treatment, the best time for this seems to be (my example) from 7.10 am to 11.15 am and from 12.30 pm to 5.00 pm. To remain mobile, please pay attention to my instructions in Chapter 6.

Cut out the daily schedule or, perhaps even better – copy it and put it somewhere in your "dining area", even if there is no food there at the moment ☺

Appendix

Time	Time	Action	Note
06.00	… o'clock	½ cup of kidney tea (for the first three weeks only)	Slowly drink cold tea
06.00	… o'clock	Hawthorn drops to stimulate cardiac performance	20-40 капель, в зависимости от комплекции
06.30	… o'clock	1-2 cups of sage tea with St. John's wort, peppermint and lemon balm	This "Breuss original sage tea" should be taken warm
07.00	… o'clock	Take a small sip of vegetable juice	Mix with saliva, swallow slowly
Throughout the day	… o'clock	1 cup (better more) of sage tea	This "Breuss original sage tea" can be taken warm or cold
	… o'clock	1 cup of cranesbill tea (herb Robert)	Drink slowly in small sips
	… o'clock	1 cup (better more) of special tea mix	Can be taken hot, warm or cold
	… o'clock	1 cup or more of marigold tea	Can be taken hot, warm or cold
In the morning	……… o'clock	Drink vegetable juice in 10-15 intakes, several sips at a time, but no more than a total of ¼ of a liter!	Drink it only if you like it, always mix with saliva!
11.30	……… o'clock	½ a cup of kidney tea (for the first three weeks only)	Slowly drink cold tea
11.30	……… o'clock	1 to 2 plates of onion broth. This broth is optional.	Before you skip onion broth, remember: it promotes healing

Appendix

Noon, 12.00	……… o'clock	Cabbage leaf compress. The compress is recommended by Breuss, but it is not a must (except in the case of stomach cancer, when it is mandatory!)	Preheated bed
In the afternoon		Drink vegetable juice in 10-15 intakes, several sips at a time but no more than a total of a ¼ of a liter!	Drink it only if you like it, always mix with saliva!
In the evening	……… o'clock	½ a cup of kidney tea (for the first three weeks only)	Before going to bed

For certain cancers, you need to drink additional herbal teas. Please note that these teas should be taken in different ways. For certain cancers, there are special procedures which should also be followed.

APPENDIX 2

Day 35

From my own experience, as well as from conversations with fellow sufferers, I am aware of the danger lurking around day 35 of cancer treatment, when the patient feels like "throwing in the towel".

On this day, one is sick and tired of everything:

- Always the same juice,
- Always the same teas,
- Always the same hawthorn drops,
- Always the same onion broth!

This does not need to be the case but such a day may come. Therefore, you should be prepared for this critical phase.

So **note**: the end of the treatment **is preceded by day 35!**

And then, it is vital to

STAY THE COURSE!!!

A warning example: A warning example: in a conversation with me, the wife of a cancer patient reported that her former neighbour also underwent The Cure. On day 37 he suddenly discontinued the treatment and demanded to be finally provided with normal food! He devoured, in defiance of common sense, a hearty meal. With the result that in a short while he was admitted to hospital. And three days later he died of internal injuries.

The autopsy showed that he had been cured of cancer! At least, there were no tumors. The man died of his own recklessness, and not of cancer, which had already been cured!

This story should be an urgent warning for you!

You should never forget the following statement by Breuss; it also applies to the critical stage of treatment:

> "The treatment can only **fail** when my instructions are not strictly adhered to **in all aspects**"

I Did It!!!
A Model Form

During the treatment, a tape measure helped me a lot; I glued it on the door of the kitchen.

42 cm long, i.e. one centimeter for each day (as with soldiers, 100 days till demobilization).

I placed zero on the top, and the number "42" - at the bottom. At the end of the first day of treatment I cut off the first centimeter, i.e., the number "42". My aim was to slowly move towards 0, meaning "**I did it!**"

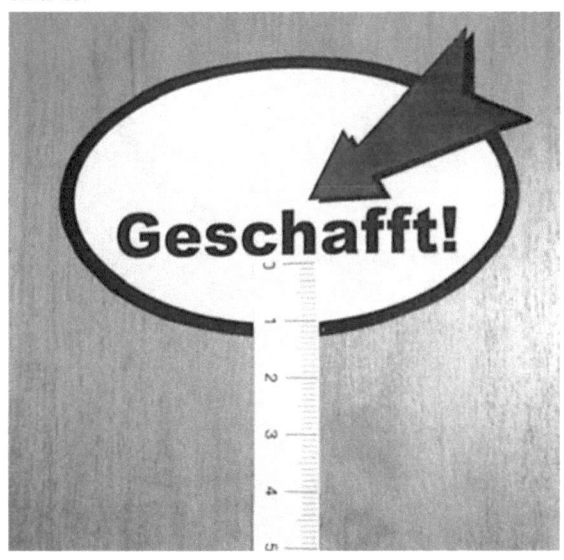

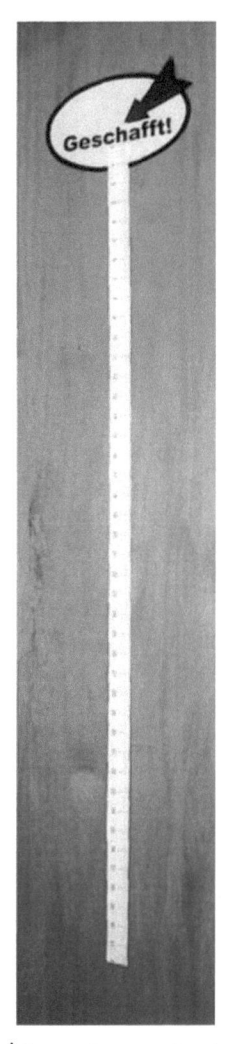

And that's how the tape looked one week before the end of the treatment, in the critical stage around day 35.

Appendix

So, my evening ritual throughout the therapy was to ceremoniously cut one centimeter from the tape. The remaining part of the treatment became another day shorter! In the top left part you can see the tape still in full length, i.e. before the end of the first day of treatment

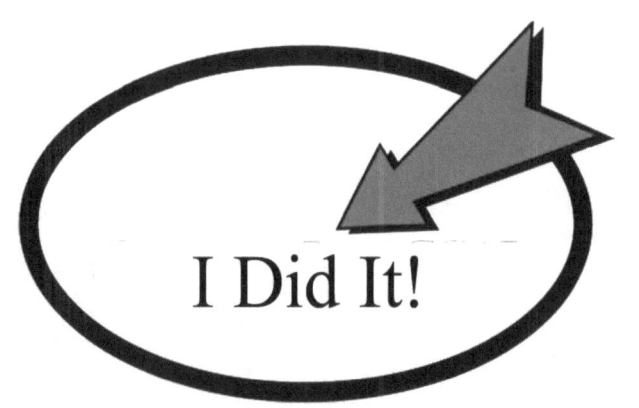

I Did It!

You can cut out this inscription ("I did it!"), or copy it and then cut it out.

APPENDIX 4

QUESTIONNAIRE
FOR COLLECTING THE BREUSS THERAPY-BASED CANCER HEALING TESTIMONIALS

Dear readers,

Many people have undergone the Rudolf Breuss cancer treatment in the last decades and recovered.

It is time to document the successes of The Cure so that it can also attract the attention of representatives of other medical practices. Among other things, it could also be done in the context of a retrospective (based on past events) study, including an anonymous (without publication of your personal data) assessment of cases when patients are reported to have been cured of cancer.

If you have already undergone the Breuss cancer treatment, or if you have decided to follow it in the near future, I would urge you to participate in this study and return this data sheet to me. You will then receive a corresponding questionnaire with the data required for the study. It goes without saying that your data will be treated anonymously and recorded exclusively for this purpose.

Rudolf Breuss writes in his book,
"Finally, I'd like to sincerely ask all reputable scientists to test my achievements scientifically…, to be with me in helping the afflicted, instead of being against me for the only reason – I am not being in a medical professional."

Appendix

Through your participation, you make sure that this natural as well as well-proven healing method is scientifically tested and receives the recognition it deserves.

In this case, conventional medical practitioners will also be able to recommend the Breuss treatment to their patients as a worthwhile therapy, and provide them with medical supervision.

Let me express my sincere appreciation for your support.

Jürgen H.R. Thomar

Jürgen H.R. Thomar

Appendix

Data Sheet for Collecting the Breuss Therapy-Based Cancer Healing Testimonials

(Please copy, complete and send to my address)

I have undergone the 42-day Breuss cancer treatment (or interrupted it) and I agree to receive a questionnaire for conducting a retrospective study.

Surname: ....

First name: ....

Street/Housenumber: ....

Zip code: ....

City/town: ....

Phone: ....

Fax: ....

E-mail: ....

Date: ....

Signature: ....

Please send via E-mail to: kontakt@thomar.net

Appendix

APPENDIX 5

TEA LABELS

Sage Tea

Put three, at the most four teaspoons, of sage in 1 liter of boiling water and **boil for exactly three minutes**. Once the sage tea has boiled for three minutes, turn off the heat and add 3-4 pinches of the "tea mix" made in advance (St. John's wort, peppermint, lemon balm). Then let everything steep for 10 minutes.
You may drink this tea as much as you want, the more the better.
Prepare its ingredients in sufficient quantity!

Tea Mix

This mixture consisting of St. John's wort, peppermint and lemon balm is added to the sage leaves and boiled for exactly three minutes.

Quantity: for one liter, you should take three to four pinches of this mix.

Marigold Tea

For a change, you can drink warm or cold marigold tea.
Preparation: one to two teaspoons (2-3 g) are poured with hot water (some 150 ml) and after 10 minutes put through a tea strainer.

Cranesbill Tea

Steep a pinch of cranesbill (herb Robert, Geranium Robertianum) in a cup of hot water (some 150 ml) for 10 minutes.
Slowly sip one cup of cold tea throughout the day.

Kidney Tea

Steep a pinch of kidney tea mixed in advance (horsetail, stinging nettle, knotgrass and St. John's wort) in a cup of hot water (some 150 ml) for 10 minutes.
Then strain out the tea leaves and set aside the liquid. Add another two cups of hot water to the tea leaves, and boil them for 10 minutes: after this, strain the tea and blend the two liquids. Drink the tea cold.
The tea volume obtained is equal to the required three half cups.

Special Tea Mix

Put a pinch of the herbs mixed in advance (plantain lance or broadleaf plantain, Iceland moss, lungwort, ground ivy, mullein and meum mutellina, if available) in a cup of hot water (approx. 150 ml) and steep for 10 minutes. Drink at least one liter of this tea each day.
You can drink as much of this tea as you want, the more the better.
So, prepare a sufficiently large amount of its ingredients!

APPENDIX 6

BIBLIOGRAPHY

- Berendes, Axel and Dr. Hofmann, Klaus: *Save Your Immune System. A Guide for Survival in Present Times* (Rette dein Immunsystem. Ein Leifaden zum Überleben in heutiger Zeit). Vier Flamingos publishing house, 1993, ISBN: 3-928306-05-07.

- Breuss, Rudolf: *Indictment* (Anklageschrift). The indictment of Rudolf Breuss is a unique complement to Breuss' "Cancer-Leukemia" book. It contains both expert evidence and counter-evidence, as well as interesting reports about "the treatment methods" of Rudolf Breuss. Breuss mail-order bookshop Walter Margreiter, format DIN A4, 32 pages.

- Breuss, Rudolf: *Natural Treatment of Cancer, Leukemia and Other Seemingly Incurable Diseases. Advice on Prevention and Treatment of Many Diseases* (Krebs/Leukämie und andere scheinbar unheilbare Krankheiten mit natürlichen Mitteln heilbar. Ratschläge zur Vorbeugung und Behandlung vieler Krankheiten), Merk publishing house, 1990, ISBN: 3-00-018407-4.

- Breuss, Rudolf: *The Breuss Cancer Cure: Advice for the Prevention and Natural Treatment of Cancer, Leukemia and Other Seemingly Incurable Diseases* (Die Breuss Krebskur, Ratschläge zur Vorbeugung und die natürliche Behandlung

Appendix

von Krebs, Leukämie und anderen scheinbar unheilbaren Krankheiten), new revised edition, Rudolf Breuss self-publishing company, Breuss mail-order bookshop Walter Margreiter, Im Hag, 23, A-6714 Nüziders/Austria, 2005, ISBN: 3-00-00429-0.

- Buchner, Elisabeth: *When Body and Feelings Play Roller Coaster... Balancing Hormones Naturally* (Wenn Körper und Seele Achterbahn spielen...Hormone natürlich ins Gleichgewicht bringen), FVB, 2000, ISBN: 3-934246-00-1.

- Carstens, Veronica, Dr. med.: *Empirical Cancer Diagnosis and Therapy* (Diagnose und Therapie von Krebs mit Mitteln der Erfahrungsheilkunde), series of publications Nature and Medicine, 2000.

- Diamond, Harvey and Marilyn: *Fit for Life* (Fit fürs Leben), Goldmann Taschenbuch Verlag publishing house, ISBN: 3-44-213533-8.

- Droz, Camille: *The Wonderful Properties of the Cabbage Leaf (Von der wunderbaren Heilwirkung des Kohlblattes)*, 1994, currently not available. For further details, please contact the Breuss mail-order bookshop Walter Margreiter, Im Hag, 23, A-6714 Nüziders/Austria, www.margreiter-buch.at, e-mail: office@ margreiter-buch.a

- Eickelen, Knut "Key": *Cancer, If Not Cured, Can Be Defeated (Krebs wenn nicht heilbar dann besiegbar)*, Books on Demand GmbH, 2009, ISBN: 9783839102558.

Appendix

- Erckenbrecht, Irmela: *Herb Spiral, Construction Manual, Herb Portraits, Recipes* (Die Kräuterspirale, Bauanleitung, Kräuterportraits, Rezepte), Pala publishing house, 2003, ISBN: 3-895 66-190-2.

- Fleig, Harald: *Healing the Spinal Column After Dorn and Breuss* (Heilen über die Wirbelsäule nach Dorn und Breuss), volume 1, B&H Fleig publishing house, 1995, ISBN: 3-9805138-0-7.

- Fleig, Harald: *Healing the Spinal Column After Breuss – Dorn – Fleig* (Heilen über die Wirbelsäule nach Breuss – Dorn – Fleig), volume 2, B&H Fleig publishing house, 1999, ISBN: 3-9805138-1-5.

- Fleig, Harald: *Healing the Spinal Column After Breuss – Dorn – Fleig* (Heilen über die Wirbelsäule nach Breuss – Dorn – Fleig), DVD, B&H Fleig publishing house, 2005, ISBN: 3-9805138-1-5.

- Griffin, Edward G.: *A World Without Cancer* (Eine Welt ohne Krebs), Kopp publishing house, 2007, ISBN: 3-938516-15-1.

- Hofer, Reinhard and Hartl, Thomas: *Cured! How People Defeated Cancer* (Geheilt! Wie Menschen den Krebs besiegten), Ueberreuter publishing house, 2012, ISBN: 978-3800072866.

Appendix

- Hofer, Reinhard: *There Are No "Incurable Diseases": How People Heal Themselves* (Es gibt kein "Unheilbar": Wie Menschen sich selbst heilen), Ueberreuter publishing house, 2012, ISBN: 978-3800075294.

- Jonsson, Bitten and Nordström, Pia: *Sugar, No, Thank You! How Sugar Is Damaging Your Body* (Zucker, nein danke! Was Zucker in Ihrem Körper anrichtet), Mosaik bei Goldmann publishing house, ISBN: 3-442-16801-5.

- *"Oncology"* (Krebsgeschehen), oncology report about the Breuss cancer treatment. The first clinical trial of this method was conducted by conventional medical practitioners at the end of 1982 in Germany; this report provides the description of the experiment (see also the "Indictment" written by Rudolf Breuss, p. 22-23), both available from Breuss mail-order bookshop Walter Margreiter, format DIN A4, 8 pages.

- Lee, John R., Dr. med., translated and supplemented by E. Buchner: *How Men Remain Strong. Natural Hormone Balance for Men* (Wie Männer stark bleiben. Natürlicher Hormonausgleich für Männer), FVB, ISBN: 3-934246-01-X.

- Lützner, Hellmut, Dr. med. and Million, Helmut: *Eating Right After Fasting* (Richtig essen nach dem Fasten), 2001, Gräfe & Unzer publishing house, ISBN: 3-77-426686-7.

- Maar, Klaus, Prof. Dr. med.: *The Truth about Prostate Cancer* (Die Wahrheit über Prostatakrebs), Kopp publishing house, 2008, ISBN: 978-3-938516-70-6.

- Nowak, Karl Walter: *Report of a Cancer Healer (A new updated edition of the book "No More Fear of Cancer")* (Der Krebsheiler Report. Aktualisierte Neuauflage des Buches "Nie mehr Angst vor Krebs"), Die Silberschnur publishing house, Caducee Edition, 2004, ISBN: 3-937464-07-7.

- Strehlow, Wighard: *The Nutrition Therapy by Hildegard von Bingen: Recipes, Cures, Diets* (Die Ernährungstherapie der Hildegard von Bingen Rezepte, Kuren, Diäten), 2003, ISBN: 3-36-303031-2.

- Strunz, Ulrich Th., Dr. med.: *Forever Young – the Success Program* (Forever Young – Das Erfolgsprogramm), dtv - paperback publications, ISBN: 3-42-3340004-5.

- Thomar, Jürgen H.R.: *That Was It – My Farewell From Cancer* (Das war's – Mein Abschied vom Krebs), 2015, Amazon, ISBN: 978-1-508416234.

- Thomar, Jürgen H.R: *Rudolf Breuss Cancer Cure Correctly Applied* (Die Breuss Krebskur richtig gemacht), 2005, private publishing house, ISBN: 3-00-016985-4.

- Thomar, Jürgen H.R.: *Practice of the Breuss Treatment* (Pratique de la Cure Breuss), 2007, Éditions Véga, Paris, ISBN: 978-2858-294701.

Appendix

- Thomar, Jürgen H.R.: *42 Day Breuss Cancer Cure* (42-dnevno zdravljenje raka po Rudolfu Breussu), Filagro Publishing, Ljubljana, ISBN: 978-9619-304518.

- Thomar, Jürgen H.R.: *Rudolf Breuss Cancer Cure Fast... Simply Ingenious* (Heilfasten nach Rudolf Breuss, einfach genial), 2007, Die Silberschnur publishing house, Caducee Edition, ISBN: 978-3-89845-191-8.

- Treben, Maria: *Health Through God's Pharmacy. Advice and Experiences with Medicinal Herbs* (Gesundheit aus der Apotheke Gottes. Ratschläge und Erfahrungen mit Heilkräutern), Wilhelm Ennsthaler publishing house, Steyr, 1980, ISBN: 3-85-0680090-8.

- Wikipedia is a free online encyclopedia created in many languages in 2001. The name "Wikipedia" is an artificia word derived from "Wiki" (a Hawaiian word meaning "quick") and "Encyclopedia".

Appendix

APPENDIX 7

ADDRESS DIRECTORY

- *Health-optimizing supplements*

  - *Bio-Strath herbal yeast* for patients in Germany: Bio-Strath herbal yeast, a manufacturer you can order from: Strath-Labor GmbH, D-93093 Donaustauf, Strathstr. 5-7, website: strath-labor.de, e-mail: strath-labor@t-online.de, phone: +40(0)9403 95090.
  Also see the information on page 129.

  - *Strath convalescence drops* for patients in Switzerland, Austria and 50 other countries worldwide: manufacturer (no factory-direct sale and no delivery to Germany): Bio-Strath AG, CH-8032 Zurich, Mühlebachstr. 38, website: www.bio-strath.ch, e-mail: info@bio-strath.ch, phone: +41(0)44-2507100.
  Also see the information on page 84 and 129.

- *Doctors specializing in therapeutic fasting*

  - *Central Association of Doctors for Natural and Alternative Medicine (ZAEN):* Am Promenadenplatz, 1, D-72250 Freudenstadt, website: www.zaen.de, e-mail: info@zaen.org, phone: +49(0)7441-918580

  - Medical Association of Fasting & Nutrition: Wilhelm-Beck-Str., 27, D-88662, Überlingen, website: www.aerztegesellschaftheilfasten.de, e-mail: info@aerztegesellschaftheilfasten.de , Secretariat, phone: +49(0)7551-8070

Appendix

- Austrian Society for Health Promotion (GGF): GGF office in Vienna, Haydnstraße 6/31, A-1060, Vienna, website: www.gesundheitsfoerderung.at, e-mail: office@gesundheitsfoerderung.at, phone: +43(01)9676650

- *Fasting centers*

  - *Samariter-Werk:* he Samariter-Werk clinic was founded by the priest, Otto Kaiser, in 1927. He is considered one of the pioneers of the fasting cure; he is mentioned in Breuss' original book. For many years, his clinics have been practicing not only traditional fasting therapy, but also the Breuss treatment.

    The Breuss fasting treatment is practiced in two centers: one is in Hörstel in Tecklenburger Land, and the other one – in Volkertshausen, not far from Lake Constance.

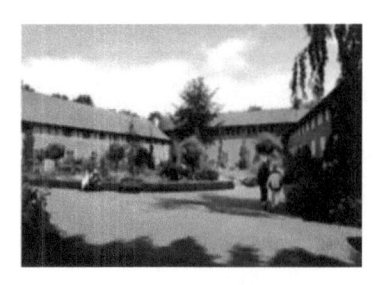

    Samaritan fasting center
    D-48477, Hörstel,
    Gravenhorster Str., 12,
    phone: +49(0) 5459-934678,
    website:
    www.fasten-zentrum.de,
    e-mail: hoerstel@fasten-zentrum.de

    Fasting center in Hörstel

Appendix

Samaritan fasting center D-78269, Volkertshausen, Samariter Weg, 7, phone: +49 (0) 7774-92900, website: www.fastenzentrum.de, e-mail: volkertshausen@fasten-zentrum.de

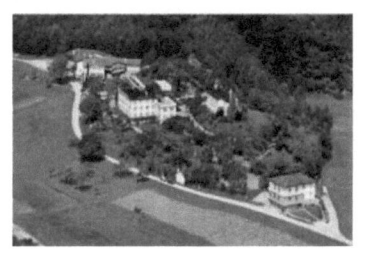

Fasting center in Volkertshausen

- *Grünemei Naturopathic Health Center: "Stilles Haus Bergfreiheit" ("Quiet House Bergfreiheit")*, A highly recommendable clinic which carries out the Breuss cancer treatment under medical supervision. A quiet and green location with the treatment performed in a responsible and prudent manner – very much in the spirit of Rudolf Breuss. Natural healing practices, fasting cure, yoga, meditation, weight correction, vegetarian food, walks, rest and recreation. Contact person: Christian T. Grünemei, homeopathic practitioner, nutritionist and expert on fasting cure. Other experienced therapists are invited to the clinic if required. Medically supervised programs are available on request. Address: D-34537, Bad Wildungen, phone 05626/999510, website: www.stilleshaus.de, e-mail: info@stilleshaus.de Also see the information on page 193.

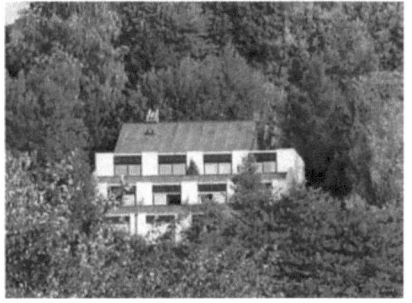

Appendix

- *Natural healing:*

  - *Brigitte and Harald Fleig, Breuss-Dorn-Fleig Spinal Care Training Center,* D-79657, Wehr, website: www.breuss-dorn-fleig-therapie.de, e-mail: harald.fleig@t-online.de, phone: +49(0) 7762-7260
  - *Homeopathic practitioner Gerhard Kerber, psycho-somatic therapy,* naturopathy, energy healing, hypnotherapy, D-88682, Salem, e-mail: G.Kerber@vdk-internet.de, phone: +49(0) 7553-829268
  - *Homeopathic practitioner Olaf Schultz-Friese, energy therapy,* colonic hydrotherapy, bioresonance therapy (MORA), D-88348 Bad-Saulgau, website: www.naturheilpraxis-bad-saulgau.de, e-mail: olaf@schultz-friese.de, phone: +49(0) 7581-2861

- *Examination of the sleeping area:*

  - *Biological examination of the sleeping area/apartment/house:* Windmöller JANatur, Dipl. Ing. Frank Windmöller, Building biology IBM, Heilenbecker Str. 161, D-58256, Ennepetal, phone: +49(0) 176-103555192, website: www.janatur-pur.com, e-mail: info@janatur-pur-com
  - *Academy for Radiation Protection and Environmental Medicine,* Unterwolfbühl 430, A-6934 Sulzberg, phone: +43(0) 5516-24671, website: www.geovital.com, e-mail: hilfe@geovital.com
  - *Association of German Dowsers,* Marianne Eger, Jacob-Jacobi-Str. 14, D-65321 Heidenrod, phone: 06775-9696236 website: www.rutengaengerverein.de, e-mail: info@rutengaengerverein.de

Appendix

- *Natural Spinal-Care® Center,* owner Michael Rau, Römerstr., 56, D-76448, Durmersheim, phone: +49(0)7245-93719-5, website: www.breuss-dorn-shop.de, e-mail: info@breuss-dorn-shop.de Also see the information on page 220

- *Drinking water treatment: Gutes Wasser GmbH,* Am Berghof, 5, D-88630, Pfullendorf, phone: +49(0) 7552/9337970, fax: 9337979, website: www.guteswasser.info, e-mail: kontakt@guteswasser.info.

  Also see the information on page 169.

Appendix

APPENDIX 8

Subject Index

A
Acid-base balance 147
Alcohol 97,132,144,155,196,215,239,243,250
Arthritis 31
Arthrosis 31

B
Bad breath 108
Bed rest 116
Beetroot 47,186,188
Biopsy 36,123,244
Blackcurrant, raspberry or pumpkin juice 114
Blood pressure 93,105,106
Body odour 108,109
Bone cancer 74
Bowel cleansing 97
Bowel movement 108,110,134
Brachytherapy 37,39,42
Bread, honey, eggs or vegetables 114
Breaking your fast 130
Breast cancer 71,242,237,240
Breuss massage 33,142
Breuss, Rudolf 267
Broth 194,195
Breuss Treatment 23,31,33,56,65,79,91,99
107,109,111,115,124,129,130,142,157,238,247,251,253,264,274
Broth of bean pods 194,195,215
Business trip 120

Appendix

C
Cabbage leaf compress 46,68,75,80
Cancer of the neck lymph nodes............73,206
Cancer risk 155,239,250
Cancer screening 241,243
Cancer treatment............
............21,26,42,43,53,55,57,59,63,70,90,119,213,222
Cancer treatment shopping list............213
Cancerous tumour............95
Cancer types............199
Candida fungus............144
Carrot 52,130,145,154,186,188,214,255
Carstens, Veronica, Doctor of Medicine............21,268,143
Celery root............188
Chemotherapy............
............61,86,90,104,115,122,125,157,227,236,249,253
Chewing gum............109
Celandine 69,73,207,217
Celandine juice 69,73,207
Celandine tea............207
Celandine tincture............207
Centaury tea............ 68,77,208
Childhood cancer............237
Choline-PET-CT............41
Coffee and cakes............97
Colon hydrotherapy............99
Compress............46,68,75,80
Constipation............106
Coxarthrosis............31
Cranesbill (Herb Robert) 67,119,200,216,226
Cranesbill tea 202,257,266
Cerebral tumor 68,72,206,217,228
Crimson (scarlet) beebalm............206
CT examination 119,35,56,94,101,116,123,226,241
Cup size 198,212

Appendix

D
Daily routine 64
Daily schedule 103,256
Data sheet for collecting Breuss therapy-based cancer........
healing testimonials... 265
Decision-making 254
Diagnostic procedures 35,122,121
DiaPat test 122
Dietary supplements 176
Distilled water 166
Dorn-therapy 33
Douwes Friedrich, Professor,
Doctor of Medicine 21,223,231,253
Drinking water 114,160,171,175,277

E
Early screening 241
Early cancer screening 243,245
Earth radiation 173
Endorphins 48,117,120
Enema 99,107
Examination of the sleeping area 276
Eyebright 68,70,205,217
Eyebright tea .... ,68,70,205
Eye cancer 68, 70,205,217

F
Faith 91,96,159
Family doctor 56,94,222,238
Fasting ....
19,29,30,48,57,58,60,61,62,89,94,120,121,130,152,229,259,273
Fasting therapy 23,30,55,57,89,120,152,169,223,229
Feedback from orthodox medical community 94
Filter technology 168
Follow-up medical check-up 35

Appendix

G
Gall bladder cancer 68,71,195,208
Gebauer, Dieter, Professor, Doctor of Medicine 4,19
Glauber's salt or Epsom salt 98
Gleason score 36
Good water 96,114,159,169,173,175
Green grocery 214
Ground ivy 203,216,266
Growths 63,79,246
Gum cancer 206

H
Happiness hormones 120
Hawthorn drops 46,95,196,257,259
Headache 110
Health-optimizing products 273
Healthy food 158
Herbal tea labels 266
Herb spiral 48,116,269
Homemade vegetable juice 154
Hormone treatment 120
Horsetail 216
Hot wraps 82
Hyperacidity 157,150

I
Iceland moss 216
If the vegetable juice doesn't taste good anymore 212
Immune system 143
Induction stove 139
Injections and radiotherapy 115
Intestinal cancer 71

Appendix

J
John's wort 65,75,81,199,201,216,226,257,266
Joint inflammation 31
Juice extractor 100
Self made Juice or buying ready-made juice? 185

K
Kidney cancer 78
Kidney tea 199
Knotgrass 199

L
Lady's mantle 207
Laryngeal cancer 240
Lemon balm 73,216
Lemon balm tea 206
Leukemia 75
Ligusticum mutellina 216,219
Linen cloth 191
Linen cloth test 189
Lip cancer 76
Liver cancer 74
Lung cancer 76
Lungwort 203,216,266

M
Mammography 243
Marigold tea 200,266
Medical check-up 121
Medical supervision 226
Metabolism 152
Microwave oven 137,182
Mineral water 164

Appendix

Most common cancer types in males 237
Most common cancer types in females 237
Mullein 203,216
Multiple sclerosis 32
Mustard seeds 98

N
Naturopathic practitioner 28
Nettle 71
New cancer cases 235
New cancer cases in Germany 236,240
Nicotine 97,147
Nitrite and nitrate levels in drinking water 165

O
Oat straw 70,78,82
Olive oil or John's wort oil 75,81
Oncology report 223
Onion soup 195
Organic (organically grown) vegetables 101,186
Organization and preparation 100
Osteoporosis 31,126,195
Ovarian cancer 71

P
Pancreatic cancer 70
Peppermint 65,201,216
Pharmacy 99,148,215
Pilot study 224
Pimpernel 206
Pimpinella magna (pimpinella major) 68,217
Pinch 204
Plantain lance and broadleaf plantain 216

Appendix

Poison in your home 100
Potato 75,132,180,189,190
Potatoes' skin tea 206
Pork 136
Preparation days 96
Preparation of herbal teas 209
Preparations 95
Preventive screening 243
Problems with buying herbal medicines 219
Prostate cancer 79
Protein 147
PSA 35
PSA level 35
Pulmonary tuberculosis 32

Q

Questionnaire for collecting Breuss therapy-based cancer healing testimonials 263

R

Radiation exposure 122
Radical surgery 40
Radiotherapy 37,115
Radish 189,214,225
Readaptation 128,132
Ready-made juice 182,186
Reheated food 156
Reverse osmosis 168

S

Sage leaves 201,202,216
Sage tea 202,200,266
Sauerkraut juice 216
Searching for the Solution 85
Selen 94,95

Appendix

Semi-vegetarianism (flexitarianism) 136
Semi-vegetarian (flexitarian) 132
Sensation of hunger 109
Serotonin 120
Shopping list 213,45,129
Silver lady's mantle tea and lady's mantle tea 207
Skin cancer 73,69,207
Smoking 114
Soil demineralization 178
Spiritual and mental preparation 95
Spleen cancer 78
Spondylarthrosis 31
St John's wort 65, 75, 81, 199,201,216, 226, 257,266
Stomach cancer 77
Stress 111,182
Support of heart function 65
Surgery 63,87
Surgery without a scalpel 63
Sweets 97,144

T

Taking control of success 121
Tap water 159,164,170,175,198
Tea with lemon 212
Teas of various strength 212
Testicular cancer 74
Thyroid cancer 80
Tongue cancer 79
Trips 119
Tumor markers 122

U

Urology 35,38
Uterine cancer 72

Appendix

V
Vegetable broth 131,195,215
Valerian tea 205,217
Vegetable juice ....
.... 46,63,70,80,97,101,113,119,154,185,190,191,192,221
Vegetable juice fasting 29,95,253
Vegetable juice with lemon 192
Vegetable juice with orange 191
Vegetable juice with sauerkraut 191
Vital substances 177

W
Waiting period 104
Water 50,
60,70,79,82,96,106,114,115,134,159,160,161,166,169,171,175,210
Water filter 168
Water veins..173
Weight loss 58
What are the benefits of ready-made juice? 186
What are the benefits of juice pressed at home? 185
White dead nettle, yellow archangel 207
Willow 68,74,79,208,217
Willow herb tea 208
Withdrawal symptoms 112
World water quality assessment 162
Wormwood tea 208,217

Printed in Poland
by Amazon Fulfillment
Poland Sp. z o.o., Wrocław